THE COMPLETE
MRCPSYCH
PART I

THE COMPLETE MRCPSYCH PART I

ASHOK G. PATEL

MRCPsych, DPM
Consultant Psychiatrist,
Fairfield Hospital, Hitchin, UK

SADGUN BHANDARI

MD, MRCPsych
Registrar,
Fairfield Hospital, Hitchin, UK

KRISHNAPILLAI BALASUBRAMANIAM

LRCP (London), MRCS (Eng.), MRCPsych
Consultant Psychiatrist,
Bedford General Hospital
Bedford and Shires Health and Care NHS Trust, UK

WB SAUNDERS COMPANY LTD

LONDON   PHILADELPHIA   TORONTO
SYDNEY   TOKYO

W. B. Saunders Company Ltd   24–28 Oval Road
London NW1 7DX, UK

The Curtis Center
Independence Square West
Philadelphia, PA 19106-3399
USA

Harcourt Brace & Company
55 Horner Avenue
Toronto, Ontario M8Z 4X6
Canada

Harcourt Brace & Company
Australia
30–52 Smidmore Street,
Marrickville, NSW 2204
Australia

Harcourt Brace & Company
Japan
Ichibancho Central Building
22–1 Ichibancho
Chiyoda-ku, Tokyo 102, Japan

A catalogue record for this book is available from the
British Library

ISBN 0–7020–2067–2

This book is printed on acid-free paper

Typeset by Intype Ltd, Wimbledon Park, London
Printed in Great Britain by Mackays of Chatham PLC,
Chatham, Kent

CONTENTS

FOREWORD

The MRCPsych is the major qualification for psychiatric trainees in the United Kingdom and this book has the important aim of assisting candidates to prepare for its Part I.

The authors are very well qualified for this task. Two of them are examiners in the Part I MRCPsych and Psychiatric Tutors, while the third is a Registrar sufficiently close to the examination to recall the issues which concern the candidates. They work in a setting of local psychiatric services, which provide their own teaching, they also were linked rotationally with London and have now forged close links with Cambridge. They have written extensively in the past on multiple choice questions and short answer questions in the MRCPsych, and have published a previous successful book on Part II of the examination. The care and attention to accurate detail which they have brought to their task are exemplary.

Books like this one serve multiple purposes. They provide a systematic way to survey the curriculum and the expectations in the examination, and then an important method of pre-testing knowledge, ordered in a more random and examination like way, to identify gaps. In these ways they are tangible aids to learning. They also provide something different but equally important – a way to practise examination technique in advance, and to deal with the potentially very real anxieties which, sadly, the examination situation can produce. Such desensitization can be very valuable, particularly in respect of MCQs, for candidates who have not had wide experience of this style of questioning in their education.

I commend the work which has gone into this carefully prepared volume, and I commend the book to its readers. I hope it may make their onerous task easier.

E. S. PAYKEL

PREFACE

This book is based on many years' experience of clinical psychiatry and teaching both under- and postgraduate students in psychiatry. It is aimed at doctors preparing for Part I of the MRCPsych examination, and their trainers, though other doctors and undergraduate students may also find it useful in learning about psychiatry. It is our hope that the readers of this book will find it both informative and challenging. We believe that its use will allow them to become familiar with both the subject matter and format of Part I, leading to success in the actual examination.

We have made every effort to verify the accuracy and appropriateness of the questions included in the book, but as in any text, some inaccuracies and ambiguities may have crept in. If in doubt, do consult other references as suggested in the Further Reading section. Readers should use this book as a study guide for self-assessment, i.e. revise the curriculum first by referring to appropriate questions in the book. Each MCQs paper consists of 50 randomly allocated questions which should give readers the 'feel' of the actual examination. An outline of the curriculum for the basic sciences is included in the book. For further details, readers should refer to the College document 'The Basic Sciences and Clinical Curricula for the MRCPsych Examinations (November 1994)'.

The Further Reading section includes a carefully selected list of books, following advice from psychiatric tutors and senior colleagues. We believe that there is some room for improvement. We have tried to cover a wide spectrum of subject matter in the book, but due to limited space it is not possible to be completely comprehensive. Constructive criticism, suggestions, new ideas and advice will be most warmly welcomed.

We would like to thank Professor Eugene Paykel, University of Cambridge, for his most helpful encouragement, suggestions, advice and his generosity in providing a Foreword.

Our sincere thanks are due to the staff of W. B. Saunders for their encouragement, advice and assistance during the preparation of the book.

It would not have been possible to produce this work without the support of our respective families.

A. G. P.
S. B.
K. B.

CONTRIBUTORS

Ashok G. Patel
MRCPsych, DPM
Consultant Psychiatrist
Fairfield Hospital
Hitchin, Hertfordshire

Sadgun Bhandari
MD, MRCPsych
Registrar in Psychiatry
Fairfield Hospital
Hitchin, Hertfordshire

Krishnapillai Balasubramaniam
LRCP, MRCS, MRCPsych
Consultant Psychiatrist
Bedford General Hospital
Bedford and Shires
Health and Care NHS Trust
Kempston Road
Bedford, Bedfordshire

FORMAT OF THE MRCPSYCH PART I EXAMINATION

MRCPsych Part I is an examination in basic clinical psychiatry with knowledge of the subject (including relevant aspects of basic science) and practical skills being of equal importance in testing the candidate's competence.

The examination consists of:

1. One Multiple Choice Questions paper
>   50 questions
>   Time allowed: 90 minutes

2. One Clinical Examination
>   Time allowed: 50 minutes to interview the patient, 10 minutes to prepare and 30 minutes with a pair of examiners

CURRICULUM FOR THE MRCPSYCH PART I EXAMINATION

The Royal College of Psychiatrists published 'The Basic Sciences and Clinical Curricula for the MRCPsych Examinations' in November 1994. The curricula are not all inclusive. For the benefit of the trainees and their trainers, we include some of the subjects in this chapter. For full details, readers should refer to the College document.

1. Psychopathology

A. *Descriptive psychopathology* (9 questions in each paper)
    For example:
    - Phenomenology of psychiatry.
    - Ways in which symptoms and signs are expressed and experienced.
    - Role of internal (personality and developmental) and external (environmental) factors in the pathogenesis of the symptoms.
    - Principles underlying the classification of the phenomena into syndromes.

B. *Dynamic/explanatory psychopathology*
    (6 questions in each paper)
    For example:
    - Freudian psychoanalytic theory.
    - Defence mechanisms.
    - Melanie Klein's theory.
    - Object relations theory.
    - Jungian concepts/theory.
    - Adler's concepts, e.g.

      – organ inferiority;
      – masculine protest.
   – Neofreudians.
   – Dreams.

C. *Cognitive and behavioural psychopathology*
   (2 questions in each paper)
   For example:
   – Principles of behaviour therapy.
   – Reinforcement.
   – Classical and operant conditioning.
   – Family therapy.
   – Escape learning.
   – Functional behavioural analysis.
   – Behaviour therapy.
   – Depression.
   – Anxiety states.
   – Phobias.
   – Eating disorders.

2. Basic psychology (4 questions in each paper)

   For example:
   – Learning theories.
   – Learning processes and aetiological formulation of
     clinical problems.
   – Stress.
   – Life events.
   – States and levels of awareness.

Social psychology
   For example:
   – Attitudes.
   – Self-psychology.

Human development
   For example:
   – Bowlby attachment theory.

- Personal (ego) identity in adolescence and adult life.
- Development of fears in childhood and adolescence with reference to age. Possible aetiological and maintenance mechanisms.

3. Classification of psychiatric disorders
(3 questions in each paper)

- DSMIIIR ⎤ Basic principles
- (DSMIV) ⎬ and 'compare and
- ICD10 ⎦ contrast' issues
- Fould's hierarchical classification.
- Research diagnostic criteria.

4. Psychiatric history-taking skills (3 questions in each paper)

- Models of psychiatric history-taking procedures.
- Importance of various aspects of history, e.g.
  - family history;
  - premorbid personality.
- Standardized interviews.
- Present state examination.
- History-taking of a special group of patients,
  e.g. depressed, psychotic, phobic, alcohol misusers, etc.

5. Mental state examination (3 questions in each paper)

- Procedures for examination of the patient's mental state.
- Importance of cognitive testing.
- Importance of insight, judgement, general knowledge etc.
- Mini Mental State examination.

6. Process of diagnosis and assessment
(2 questions in each paper)

- Establishing satisfactory working relationship with the patient.
- Eliciting of accurate information.
- Integrating the information obtained in clinical assessment.
- The recognition of the need for further examination, information and/or investigations.

7. Aetiology of psychiatric disorders
(2 questions in each paper)

- Role of predisposing, precipitating, perpetuating and maintaining factors.
- Role of learning experiences, e.g.
  - separation anxiety;
  - bereavement;
  - loss of parents, spouses, siblings etc.
- Role of psychodynamic theories.
- Role of physical disorders.

8. Basic clinic psychopharmacology (4 questions in each paper)

- Main groups of psychotropic drugs, e.g.
  - anxiolytics;
  - antipsychotics;
  - antidepressives;
  - sedatives/hypnotics;
  - anticonvulsants, including carbamazepine.
- Drug action/mechanism of action.
- Adverse drug reactions: early and late, common and rare, including those within therapeutic range.
- Drug interactions.

- Clinical use of drugs.
- Systems of drug classifications.
- Basic principles of pharmacokinetics and pharmacodynamics.
- Pharmacological principles relevant to the prescribing of psychotropic drugs.

9. Neurosciences

A. *Neuroanatomy* (3 questions in each paper)
   For example:
   - Brain.
   - Spinal cord.
   - Peripheral nervous system.
   - Limbic system.
   - Basal ganglia.
   - Papez circuit.
   - Hypothalamic nuclei.
   - Blood supply of brain.
   - Blood–brain barrier.
   - Reticular activating system.
   - Neocortex.
   - Posterior columns.
   - Lower and upper motor neurones.

B. *Neuropathology/clinical neurology*
   (3 questions in each paper)
   For example:
   - Principal neuropathological changes in
     - degenerative disorders;
     - cerebrovascular disorders;
     - other conditions which may be referred to psychiatrists.

C. *Neurophysiology* (3 questions in each paper)
   For example:
   - Sensory and autonomic nervous systems.
   - EEG – normal and abnormal.

- Sleep and its disorders.
- Evoked potentials.
- Action potential.
- Anomalous rectification.

D. *Neurochemistry* (2 questions in each paper)
   For example:
   - Neurotransmitters/ neuroreceptors.
   - Pathways of neurotransmitters.
   - Role of neurotransmitters in psychiatric disorders.
   - GABA shunt.
   - Calcium channels.
   - Endorphins.
   - Brain lipids.
   - Neuropeptides.

E. *Neurological examination* (1 question in each paper)

OUTLINE OF THE MCQS PAPER

1. **Psychopathology**
   A. Descriptive psychopathology
   B. Dynamic/explanatory psychopathology
   C. Cognitive and behavioural psychopathology

2. **Basic psychology, social psychology and human development**

3. **Classification of psychiatric disorders**

4. **Psychiatric history-taking skills**

5. **Mental state examination**

6. **Process of diagnosis and assessment**

7. **Aetiology of psychiatric disorders**

8. **Basic clinical psychopharmacology**

9. **Neurosciences**
   A. Neuroanatomy
   B. Neuropathology/clinical neurology
   C. Neurophysiology
   D. Neurochemistry
   E. Neurological examination

THE MCQS PAPERS: GUIDELINES

Each question consists of a stem followed by five suggested answers. The candidates are asked to indicate whether each answer is true or false or to state 'Don't know'. There is no restriction on the number of true or false answers in any individual question. However, it is believed that approximately 50% of answers are true and the rest are false.

Negative marking

The answers correctly identified as true or false receive a mark of +1. Those marked as 'Don't know' receive a zero mark, while incorrectly identified answers (that is, true as false and false as true answers) receive a penalty mark of −1. Guesswork is therefore not rewarding and may be damaging.

Develop a clear understanding of various terms used in these questions as well as the format and style of the question.

All the answers are independent of one another; in other words, one cannot derive a clue about an answer from another.

The first impression is often the best, so beware of making changes unless they are based on insight.

Read each paper carefully and answer the questions under strict examination conditions. This will help you to identify your strengths and weaknesses. Having done this, refer to the given answers and explanations.

If you understand the stem of the question thoroughly, it is worthwhile making a guess, but if you are unsure it is advisable not to guess.

Practise according to these principles in order to assess your knowledge as follows:

(a) Don't know but would guess.
(b) Don't know and would not guess.

Two methods to use to answer the MCQs papers

It is a matter of choice for each examinee to use one of these methods, but we recommend the first method in the examination.

1. Mark all the answers as 'T' for true, 'F' for false or 'D' for 'Don't know' on the question paper. Then carefully transfer all the answers onto the answer sheet provided. Make sure that all the answers are marked in the correct boxes.

   We believe that it is much easier to transfer the answers to the answer sheet than to answer the questions and mark the answer sheet when there is a shortage of time. This technique may also allow some spare time to revisit outstanding queries in the paper.

2. Answer the questions as you go; read and mark them on the answer sheet immediately. Repeat the process until you reach the last question. It may be that you will find some questions difficult to answer correctly; if so, leave them and proceed to the next question. Revisit the unanswered questions.

There is no minimum or maximum number of answers to the questions for a pass mark. We would advise you to answer confidently as many questions as you can.

Explanation of Terms Used in MCQs

There is a consensus that the following terms have the following implied meanings:

1. **Occurs:**
   Makes no statement about frequency (i.e. a recognized occurrence).

2. **Recognized:**
   Has been reported as a feature or association.

3. **Characteristic or typical:**
   Features that occur so often as to be of some diagnostic significance and whose absence might lead to some doubt being cast on diagnosis.

4. **Essential/diagnostic feature:**
   Must occur to make a diagnosis.

5. **Specific or pathognomonic:**
   Features that occur in the named disease and no other.

6. **Can be or may be:**
   It is recognized (i.e. reported) as occurring.

7. **Commonly, frequently, is likely or often:**
   Imply a rate of occurrence greater than 50%.

8. **Always or never:**
   Suggest that there are no recognized exceptions.

9. **Particularly associated:**
   The association is significant in samples with sufficient numbers.

10. **Exclusively:**
   Features that occur in the named condition and no others.

11. **Invariably:**
   Implies the occurrence of a feature without a shadow of doubt.

12. **Only:**
   Singles out a feature or a condition.

13. **Include:**
   Like 'occurs' makes no mention of frequency.

14. **Majority:**
   Means 50% or more.

15. **Implicit:**
   Implied though not plainly expressed, virtually contained.

16. **Explicit:**
   Expressly stated, leaving nothing merely implied, stated in detail.

17. **Usually:**
   60% or more.

PAPER 1

1. *Characteristic pathological features of dementia in Alzheimer's disease type 2 include:*
   (a) Neuritic plaques. *L before 65yrs*
   (b) Reactive astrocytosis.
   (c) Hirano bodies.
   (d) Lewy bodies.
   (e) Amyloid angiopathy.

2. *Catatonia:*
   (a) Occurs exclusively in schizophrenia.
   (b) Is a common presentation in conversion disorders.
   (c) Includes the phenomenon of 'Mitmachen'.
   (d) Includes the phenomenon of 'Gedankenlautwerden'.
   (e) Was first described by Kasanin.
   L schizoaffective

3. *Blood supply of the optic radiation is provided by:*
   (a) Anterior communicating artery.
   (b) Central branches of anterior cerebral artery.
   (c) Posterolateral branches of posterior cerebral artery.
   (d) Anterior choroidal artery.
   (e) Posterior cerebral artery.

4. *In dynamic psychopathology, paranosic gain:* *⌐1° gain*
   (a) Is environmental which can be shaped by the culture and society.
   (b) Is the immediate consequence of defence processes.
   (c) Is a means of discharging tension created by intrapsychic conflicts.
   (d) Is a temporary freedom from work demands.
   (e) Results in impulse control.

5. *The following statements about risperidone are correct:*
   (a) It is a benzisoxazole derivative.
   (b) It acts as an antagonist at D2 receptors.
   (c) It acts as agonist at S2 receptors.
   (d) It has no actions on the noradrenergic and histaminergic receptors.
   (e) It has an increased liability to produce extrapyramidal symptoms.

6. *Characteristic features of obsessional personality include:*
   (a) Parsimony.
   (b) Lack of adaptability to new situations.
   (c) Obstinacy.
   (d) Indecision.
   (e) Persistent difficulties in establishing a sexual relationship.

7. *The following statements about dynamic psychotherapy are correct:*
   (a) It aims to offer an opportunity for a transference relationship to grow and develop.
   (b) It inevitably contains a behavioural modification component.
   (c) It is mainly concerned with neurotic symptoms.
   (d) It aims to offer an opportunity for countertransference to grow and develop.
   (e) It involves exclusive analysis of the patient's characteristic defence mechanisms.

8. *Objective evidence of a patient's feelings during an interview can be divulged by:*
   (a) Observing the facial expressions.
   (b) The motor behaviour.
   (c) The patient's stated feelings.
   (d) The pattern of speech.
   (e) Emotional behaviour during the interview.

9. *The following drugs cause fast activity on the electroencephalogram:*
    (a) Chlordiazepoxide.
    (b) Carbamazepine.
    (c) Chlorpromazine.
    (d) Fluoxetine.
    (e) Lithium carbonate.

10. *The following factors have been associated with increased incidence of schizophrenia:*
    (a) Perinatal complications.
    (b) Conception during winter months.
    (c) Birth injury.
    (d) Adoption at birth by a schizophrenic mother.
    (e) Identical twins.

11. *The recognized ego defence mechanisms in obsessive compulsive disorder include:*
    (a) Denial.
    (b) Magic doing and undoing.
    (c) Suppression.
    (d) Reaction formation.
    (e) Isolation.

12. *The following concepts regarding Freud's model of the mind are correct:*
    (a) The id is the most destructive element of the mind.
    (b) The ego functions by a conscious process.
    (c) The id is the primary source of libidinal energy.
    (d) The superego functions by means of secondary process thinking.
    (e) The id functions entirely by an unconscious process.

13. *Occlusion of the dominant middle cerebral artery at its origin causes*:
    (a) Contralateral exaggerated deep reflexes.
    (b) Difficulty in understanding both written and spoken speech.
    (c) Contralateral hemiplegia.
    (d) Positive Babinski's sign.
    (e) Partial ipsilateral facial awareness.

14. *The patient who is breast feeding should avoid the following drugs*:
    (a) Amitriptyline.
    (b) Sulpiride.
    (c) Carbamazepine.
    (d) Lithium carbonate.
    (e) Sertraline.

15. *Typical features of pathological grief reaction include the following*:
    (a) The bereaved searches for the deceased person.
    (b) Visual hallucinations.
    (c) Denial.
    (d) Auditory hallucinations.
    (e) Resurrection of the deceased person's last illness.

16. *Physiological changes which occur after ECT include*:
    (a) EEG changes usually persist for over a week.
    (b) A rise in serum prolactin shortly after the treatment.
    (c) A fall in plasma cortisol within an hour of the treatment.
    (d) An initial bradycardia and subsequent tachycardia.
    (e) A decrease in cerebral circulation.

17. *Classification of the following psychiatric disorders is based on aetiology*:
    (a) Delirium tremens.
    (b) Wilson's disease.
    (c) Korsakoff's disease.
    (d) Alzheimer's disease.
    (e) Briquet's syndrome.

18. *In hysterical conversion syndrome, the symptoms*:
    (a) Reduce conscious anxiety.
    (b) Only occur in an hysterical personality.
    (c) Are mediated via the autonomic nervous *peripheral* system.
    (d) Are symbolic representations of intrapsychic conflicts.
    (e) Disappear as soon as the primary gain is achieved.

19. *Significant memory impairment is caused by the lesions in*:
    (a) Hippocampus.
    (b) Broca's area.
    (c) Mamillary bodies.
    (d) Fornix.
    (e) Anterior perforated substance.

20. *Characteristic features of posterior column lesion include*:
    (a) Loss of conscious proprioception.
    (b) Loss of pain sensation.
    (c) Loss of discrimination touch.
    (d) Loss of sensation of body image.
    (e) Cerebellar ataxia.

21. *According to Freud's psychoanalytic theory*:
    (a) The id functions by means of primary process thinking.
    (b) The ego functions by means of tertiary process thinking.
    (c) The id aims at immediate release of tension without regard to the consequences.
    (d) The superego is the conscience of the individual.
    (e) The id obeys the reality principle.

22. *The clinical effects of stimulation of dopamine receptors include*:
    (a) Sedation.
    (b) Nausea and vomiting.
    (c) Diuresis.
    (d) Dyskinesias.
    (e) Drive.

23. *Typical features of compensation neurosis include*:
    (a) Ultimate resolution of the symptoms when the claim is settled.
    (b) Frontal headaches.
    (c) Fainting attacks.
    (d) Severe difficulties with sleep.
    (e) Seeking financial compensation after sustaining a relatively major injury.

24. *With regard to techniques used during a psychiatric interview*:
    (a) Reflection refers to the exact repetition of what the patient has said.
    (b) Direct questions seek information of a non-specific nature.
    (c) Confrontation refers to a technique in which further information and explanation are elicited from a patient.
    (d) Silence should be avoided at all possible cost.
    (e) Recapitulation should be used at the beginning of the interview.

25. *Haptic hallucinations*:
    (a) Refer to cutaneous perceptions of vague tingling.
    (b) Occur in schizophrenia.
    (c) Refer to sensations of temperature change.
    (d) Are generally not of any diagnostic significance.
    (e) Refer to a feeling of movements just below the skin.

26. *With regard to the classification of psychiatric disorders*:
    (a) Most psychiatric disorders have pathognomonic symptoms.
    (b) The symptoms used to define an illness can be reliably elicited.
    (c) Diagnosis is usually based on a group of symptoms.
    (d) External validity of most psychiatric diagnoses is high.
    (e) One based on psychodynamic principles would be the most reliable.

27. *In exposure therapy:*
    (a) Graded hierarchies are no longer used.
    (b) Exposure need not be repeated.
    (c) The first task should not provoke any anxiety.
    (d) Exposure should be prolonged.
    (e) Interval between practice sessions should be long.

28. *Recognized causes of papilloedema include:*
    (a) Central retinal vein thrombosis.
    (b) Hypoparathyroidism.
    (c) Cavernous sinus thrombosis.
    (d) Hypercapnia.
    (e) Temporal arteritis.

29. *Auditory hallucinations in clear consciousness occur in:*
    (a) Atropine poisoning.
    (b) Amphetamine abuse.
    (c) Alcohol abuse.
    (d) Cocaine abuse.
    (e) Mushroom poisoning.

30. *Visual accommodation may be adversely affected by:*
    (a) Chlordiazepoxide.
    (b) Dothiepin.
    (c) Sertraline.
    (d) Trazodone.
    (e) Benztropine.

31. *Purkinje cells:*
    (a) Send axons to cerebellar nuclei.
    (b) Receive direct innervation from mossy fibres.
    (c) Contain GABA in high concentration.
    (d) Characteristically degenerate in Pierre-Marie's hereditary cerebellar ataxia.
    (e) Send efferents to the lateral vestibular nucleus.

32. *Eidetic images*:
   (a) Are visual hallucinations.
   (b) Have never been perceived in relation to a real object.
   (c) May be thought of as 'photographic memory'.
   (d) Are a form of exterocepted visual hallucinations.
   (e) Can be called up and terminated by voluntary effort.

33. *The interviewer's behaviour during an interview which could lead to an inadequate disclosure by the patient include*:
   (a) Normalization.
   (b) Premature reassurance.
   (c) Open-ended questioning.
   (d) Switching.
   (e) False reassurance.

34. *Transference*:
   (a) Is an experience of a feeling toward a person that does not befit the person but belongs to another person in the past.
   (b) Is interpreted thoroughly in supportive psychotherapy.
   (c) Is a response to countertransference.
   (d) Can be differentiated from non-transference by its degree and character.
   (e) Is thoroughly analysed in analytic psychotherapy.

35. *The following statements about neuritic plaques are correct*:
   (a) They are characteristic features of Alzheimer's disease.
   (b) Their number correlates with the degree of intellectual decline.
   (c) They occur in dementia pugilistica.
   (d) They are diagnostic features of punch-drunk syndrome.
   (e) They are intracellular brain structures.

36. *In the first month of bereavement, morbid rather than normal grief is indicated by*:
    (a) Persistent denial of loss.
    (b) Recurrent panic attacks.
    (c) Self-blame.
    (d) Recurrent nightmares involving the deceased.
    (e) Searching behaviour.

37. *Factors which significantly increase the risk of suicide in a schizophrenic patient include*:
    (a) Thought echo.
    (b) Presence of akathisia.
    (c) Fear of mental disorientation.
    (d) Unemployment.
    (e) High premorbid educational attainment.

38. *The cognitive behavioural model of depression*:
    (a) Gives primacy to emotional states that give rise to cognitions.
    (b) Was influenced by the work of Albert Ellis.
    (c) Uses the concept of schemas.
    (d) Includes Eysenck's depressive triad.
    (e) Suggests that events play no part in the occurrence of depression.

39. *Reciting the months of the year in reverse order*:
    (a) Is a test for short-term memory.
    (b) Is a test for general knowledge.
    (c) Is a test for long-term memory.
    (d) Is usually impaired in agoraphobia.
    (e) Is usually unimpaired in delirium tremens.

40. *Overeating is a recognized feature of*:
    (a) Anorexia nervosa.
    (b) Agoraphobia.
    (c) Social phobia.
    (d) Bulimia nervosa.
    (e) Depression.

41. *Treatment with the following drugs causes significant weight gain*:
    (a) Fluoxetine.
    (b) Carbamazepine.
    (c) Moclobemide.
    (d) Diazepam.
    (e) Risperidone.

42. *The following are types of schedules of reinforcement*:
    (a) Fixed interval schedule.
    (b) Fixed reinforcement schedule.
    (c) Variable reinforcement schedule.
    (d) Fixed ratio schedule.
    (e) Variable ratio schedule.

43. *The following statements about brief dynamic psychotherapy are correct*:
    (a) Focalization of the conflict is an essential feature.
    (b) Termination date is set in advance in all types of brief dynamic psychotherapy.
    (c) It is most helpful in circumscribed neurotic problems.
    (d) Malan and Horowitz are the leading practitioners of brief dynamic psychotherapy.
    (e) Its main indication is patients with difficulties in personal relationships.

44. *Acetylcholine is a principal neurotransmitter at*:
    (a) Presynaptic sympathetic ganglia.
    (b) Spinal Renshaw cell.
    (c) Presynaptic parasympathetic ganglia.
    (d) Mesolimbic tract.
    (e) Neuromuscular junction.

45. *In cognitive theory, the term 'cognition' is used in naming the following phenomena*:
    (a) Cognitive events.
    (b) Cognitive attitudes.
    (c) Cognitive beliefs.
    (d) Cognitive processes.
    (e) Cognitive structures.

46. *Clinical features of normal weight bulimia include:*
    (a) Abdominal striae.
    (b) Lanugo hair.
    (c) Bradycardia.
    (d) Erosion of tooth enamel.
    (e) Calluses on the fingers.

47. *Reciting the months of the year in reverse order:*
    (a) Is a test for concentration.
    (b) Can be impaired in generalized anxiety disorder.
    (c) Is variable depending upon the intellect level.
    (d) Can be impaired in depression.
    (e) Can be normal in early dementia.

48. *Regarding ICD10:*
    (a) It categorizes alcohol abuse separately from abuse of other drugs.
    (b) The number of categories containing the diagnosis of depression has been nearly halved in comparison with ICD9.
    (c) It continues to distinguish between psychoses and neuroses.
    (d) The final text was produced after field trials.
    (e) The field trials were a lot more extensive than the ones used for ICD9.

49. *Clinical features of syringomyelia include:*
    (a) Loss of sensitivity to pain.
    (b) Loss of sensitivity to temperature.
    (c) Loss of sensitivity to touch.
    (d) Ulcers on the fingers.
    (e) Bell's palsy.

50. *Night terrors:*
    (a) Occur in stage IV of orthodox sleep.
    (b) Are genetically linked to sleepwalking.
    (c) Occur in the first half of the night.
    (d) Are associated with slow alpha rhythm.
    (e) Occur exclusively in REM sleep.

PAPER 2

1. *In comparison with DSMIIIR, ICD10*:
   (a) Includes post-psychotic depression under affective disorders.
   (b) Has an extended classification of short lasting psychotic disorders.
   (c) Includes schizotypal disorders under schizophrenia.
   (d) Extends the age of onset of autism to 48 months.
   (e) Uses narcissistic personality as an inclusion term for passive aggressive personality disorder.

2. *Hyperphagia characteristically occurs in*:
   (a) Klüver–Bucy syndrome.
   (b) Kleine–Levin syndrome.
   (c) Anorexia nervosa.
   (d) Bulimia nervosa.
   (e) Bipolar affective disorder.

3. *The following statements about schedules of reinforcement are correct*:
   (a) A smooth pattern of behaviour is found with a variable-ratio schedule.
   (b) Rate of response decreases following reinforcement in a fixed-ratio schedule.
   (c) In a variable-ratio schedule, rate of response tends to be very rapid.
   (d) 'Scalloping' occurs in a fixed-interval schedule.
   (e) In a fixed-interval schedule, the number of responses increases in inverse proportion to the duration of the interval.

4. *Psychosexual history in a severely depressed married patient should include*:
   (a) Repeated masturbation.
   (b) Recent change in sexual behaviour.
   (c) Number of previous sexual partners.
   (d) Recent change in sexual desire.
   (e) Latent homosexuality.

5. *Clinical features of Bell's palsy include*:
   (a) Facial paralysis.
   (b) Ptosis of eyelid.
   (c) Drooling of saliva from the corner of the mouth.
   (d) Hyperacusis.
   (e) Trigeminal neuralgia.

6. *The valid tests of orientation in a delirious patient include*:
   (a) Giving correct date of birth.
   (b) Ability to perform mental arithmetic.
   (c) Awareness of the role of the interviewer.
   (d) Correct awareness of passage of time.
   (e) Giving correct address.

7. *Catatonic phenomenon includes*:
   (a) Posturing.
   (b) Lhermitte's sign.
   (c) Negativism.
   (d) Command automatism.
   (e) Excitement.

8. *Characteristic features of pseudobulbar palsy include*:
   (a) Exaggerated jaw jerk.
   (b) Emotional lability.
   (c) Wasting of tongue.
   (d) Fasciculation of facial muscles.
   (e) Dysphonia.

9. *Depersonalization–derealization syndrome is significantly associated with*:
   (a) 'Near-death' experiences.
   (b) Phobic disorders.
   (c) Obsessive compulsive disorder.
   (d) Sensory deprivation.
   (e) Depression.

10. *G-protein-coupled receptors*:
   (a) Have seven transmembrane spanning sites.
   (b) Have five intracellular loops.
   (c) Have an extracellular C-terminal.
   (d) Have an intracellular N-terminal.
   (e) Belong to several distinct superfamilies of central nervous system receptors.

11. *The cognitive model of anxiety states that*:
   (a) Events are responsible for anxiety.
   (b) People's interpretations of events are responsible for anxiety.
   (c) Interpretation of the perceived loss is responsible for anxiety.
   (d) Cognitions relate to perceived danger.
   (e) The patient's responses are appropriate to the situations in which they occur.

12. *An abnormal EEG is commonly found in the following*:
   (a) Subdural haematoma.
   (b) Narcolepsy.
   (c) Night terrors.
   (d) Antisocial personality disorder.
   (e) Cerebral abscess.

13. *In supportive psychotherapy*:
   (a) The therapist actively offers advice.
   (b) Negative transference is avoided as far as possible.
   (c) Dream interpretation is an essential part.
   (d) Transference neurosis is an essential part.
   (e) The regulation of the relationship between patient and therapist is important.

14. *The following statements about ICD10 are correct*:
    (a) It is a multiaxial classification.
    (b) It is mainly a classification system of adult psychiatric disorders.
    (c) It provides practical guidance about psychiatric diagnosis.
    (d) It does not use the word 'hysteria' at all.
    (e) It contains only psychiatric disorders.

15. *Good diagnostic interviewing technique includes the following*:
    (a) Maintaining constant eye contact.
    (b) Asking directly about feelings.
    (c) Avoiding uncomfortable silences.
    (d) Deferring questions about alcohol use until a second interview.
    (e) Avoiding taking notes during the interview.

16. *Reversible causes of cognitive impairment include*:
    (a) Uraemia.
    (b) Parkinson's disease.
    (c) Depression.
    (d) Alcoholism.
    (e) Benzodiazepines.

17. *Characteristic features of Alzheimer's disease include*:
    (a) Localized atrophy of frontal cortex.
    (b) Widening of sulci.
    (c) Loss of neurones in the basal nucleus of Meynert.
    (d) Loss of dopamine neurones from the basal nucleus.
    (e) Innumerable amyloid plaques and neurofibrillary tangles.

18. *Common side-effects of tricyclic antidepressant drugs include*:
    (a) Fine tremor.
    (b) Insomnia.
    (c) Nausea.
    (d) Constipation.
    (e) Skin rash.

19. *The pyramidal pathway*:
   (a) Passes through the tegmentum in mesencephalon.
   (b) Decussates completely at medulla oblongata.
   (c) Characteristically degenerates in tabes dorsalis.
   (d) Sends efferents to ventrolateral nucleus of thalamus.
   (e) Terminates in Renshaw cells in the ventral horn of the spinal cord.

20. *Inability to sit in an interview*:
   (a) Is a diagnostic feature of hypomania.
   (b) Occurs in absence of psychiatric illness.
   (c) Does not occur in Alzheimer's disease.
   (d) Is a characteristic feature of generalized anxiety disorder.
   (e) May be due to akathisia.

21. *Neurofibrillary tangles are characteristically seen in*:
   (a) Down's syndrome.
   (b) Huntington's chorea.
   (c) Pick's disease.
   (d) Punch-drunk syndrome.
   (e) Multi-infarct dementia.

22. *Depersonalization*:
   (a) Is associated with increased anxiety.
   (b) Is usually associated with derealization.
   (c) Lasts for a short period in normal people.
   (d) Is a characteristic feature of depression.
   (e) Is frequently associated with panic attacks.

23. *Penile erection*:
   (a) Occurs in NREM sleep.
   (b) Is impaired in severe depression.
   (c) Is exaggerated in generalized anxiety disorder.
   (d) Is decreased by anticholinergic agents.
   (e) Is facilitated by the sacral roots of parasympathetic nerves.

24. *In phobias:*
    (a) The main defence mechanism is similar to that found in conversion disorder.
    (b) Repression is the first defence mechanism employed by the patient.
    (c) Different mechanisms operate in agoraphobia and social phobia.
    (d) Unconscious conflict is oedipal.
    (e) Isolation and undoing are important defence mechanisms operating in social phobia.

25. *Common side-effects of selective serotonin reuptake inhibitor drugs include:*
    (a) Vomiting.
    (b) Headache.
    (c) Drowsiness.
    (d) Dry mouth.
    (e) Diarrhoea.

26. *Sigmund Freud:*
    (a) Is considered as the father of ego psychology.
    (b) Put forward the id, ego and superego as a topographical model of the mind.
    (c) Described Oedipal complex in girls and Electra complex in boys.
    (d) Considered the id to be a completely unconscious intrapsychic conflict.
    (e) Described oral and anal as the first two stages of psychosexual development.

27. *Somatic manifestations of psychiatric disorders:*
    (a) Occur more commonly in the elderly.
    (b) Occur more commonly in children.
    (c) Occur more commonly in higher social class.
    (d) Occur more commonly in Eastern countries.
    (e) Are culturally determined.

28. *The ionotropic receptors:*
    (a) Are part of the superfamily of G-protein-coupled receptors.
    (b) Include the NMDA receptors.
    (c) Contain a central ion channel.
    (d) Involve charged particles (ions) which pass through the ionophore to enter the neurone.
    (e) On stimulation cause rapid changes in neuronal excitability.

29. *Neurotic defence mechanisms include:*
    (a) Displacement.
    (b) Rationalization.
    (c) Somatization.
    (d) Projection.
    (e) Splitting.

30. *The neocortex consists of:*
    (a) Broca's motor speech area.
    (b) Hippocampus.
    (c) Primary olfactory area.
    (d) Superior temporal gyrus.
    (e) Cingulate gyrus.

31. *The following statements about mental state examination are correct:*
    (a) When testing short-term memory, a 5 minute interval between presenting information and asking for its recall is sufficient.
    (b) If the serial sevens test cannot be performed reliably, digit span will be a reliable test of short-term memory.
    (c) The months of the year in reverse order is a satisfactory substitute for the serial sevens test.
    (d) Misidentification of the date with an error of 2 days is a sensitive indicator of disorientation.
    (e) Poor recall of the Babcock sentence is a reliable indicator of the presence of organic brain disorder.

32. *Recognized features of REM sleep include*:
   (a) Penile erection.
   (b) Vivid dreams.
   (c) Nightmares.
   (d) Loss of muscle tone.
   (e) Increased alpha activity in the electroencephalograph.

33. *Characteristic features of clouding of consciousness include*:
   (a) Partial amnesia on recovery.
   (b) Disorientation for time, place and person.
   (c) Visual hallucinations.
   (d) Perplexed mood.
   (e) Restlessness.

34. *The correct statements regarding treatment with neuroleptic drugs include*:
   (a) Akathisia usually occurs within first 5 days of treatment.
   (b) Elderly females are more prone to extrapyramidal side-effects.
   (c) Young males are more prone to tardive dyskinesia.
   (d) Akathisia occurs less frequently than dystonia.
   (e) Concomitant anti-Parkinsonian drug should not be prescribed routinely.

35. *Self-psychology*:
   (a) Is derived from the seminal writings of Kernberg.
   (b) Stresses how external relationships help maintain self-esteem and self-cohesion.
   (c) Deals with mirror-transference and idealizing-transference.
   (d) Is not of any use in narcissistic patients.
   (e) Is the same as object relations theory.

36. *Significant memory loss occurs with*:
   (a) Temporal lobe lesions.
   (b) Lesions of the uncus.
   (c) Lesions in the amygdala.
   (d) Microscopic haemorrhages in the mamillary bodies.
   (e) Left parietal lobe lesions.

37. *The characteristic features of catatonia include*:
    (a) Echolalia.
    (b) Cataplexy.
    (c) Psychological pillow.
    (d) Stereotypies.
    (e) Echopraxia.

38. *The following statements about object relations theory are correct*:
    (a) It is fundamentally similar to ego psychology.
    (b) Melanie Klein is usually considered as the founder of the object relations movement.
    (c) It encompasses the transformation of interpersonal relationships into internalized representations of relationships.
    (d) Fairburn coined the term 'good enough mothering'.
    (e) Klein described paranoid and depressive positions.

39. *Disturbances in the passage of time occur in the following*:
    (a) Major depression.
    (b) Chronic fatigue syndrome.
    (c) Depersonalization.
    (d) Intoxication with LSD.
    (e) Mania.

40. *Mowrer's two-step conditioning process*:
    (a) Was hypothesized to explain obsessions.
    (b) Forms the basis for systematic desensitization.
    (c) Consists of the first step which refers to the development of fears that occurred in early childhood.
    (d) Uses concepts of both classical and operant conditioning.
    (e) Consists of the second step which refers to the reinforcing aspect of avoidance.

41. *The following statements about ICD10 are correct*:
    (a) It is developed by the World Health Organization.
    (b) It is extensively used in Europe.
    (c) It uses separate coding for severity.
    (d) It is applicable to hospital patients only.
    (e) It forms the basis of statistical information in the United Kingdom.

42. *Depressed mood in a patient may be suggested by*:
    (a) Drooping of the angle of the mouth.
    (b) Raised medial aspect of the eyebrow.
    (c) Talking in a soft voice.
    (d) Using only limited vocabulary.
    (e) Avoidance of eye contact.

43. *Absent knee and ankle jerks are characteristically seen in*:
    (a) Huntington's chorea.
    (b) Punch-drunk syndrome.
    (c) Guillain–Barré syndrome.
    (d) Motor neurone disease.
    (e) Alzheimer's disease.

44. *Hypochondriacal delusions are a recognized feature in*:
    (a) Schizophrenia.
    (b) Illness phobia.
    (c) Social phobia.
    (d) Severe depressive illness.
    (e) Somatoform disorder.

45. *Cognitive behavioural aspects of depression include*:
    (a) Object loss.
    (b) Denial.
    (c) Learned helplessness.
    (d) Diminished social skills.
    (e) Scapegoating.

46. *Lower motor neurones*:
    (a) Lie in the anterior grey column of spinal cord.
    (b) Innervate the muscles of the hand.
    (c) Are selectively destroyed in poliomyelitis.
    (d) Lie in the posterior grey column of spinal cord.
    (e) Are attacked by varicella zoster.

47. *Learned helplessness*:
    (a) Was first described by Seligman.
    (b) Has been used in experiments with animals.
    (c) Is frequently seen in depression.
    (d) Occurs when reward is no longer contingent on the desired behaviour.
    (e) Is associated with social phobia.

48. *Drugs contraindicated in hepatic failure include*:
    (a) Carbamazepine.
    (b) Chlorpromazine.
    (c) Fluvoxamine.
    (d) Paroxetine.
    (e) Lofepramine.

49. *According to psychodynamic theories the following statements about depression are correct*:
    (a) It has been linked to the depressive position by Melanie Klein.
    (b) It is raised because of introjection of a lost object according to ego psychology.
    (c) Aggression is considered as pivotal to the understanding of depression by Bibring.
    (d) It is similar to mourning.
    (e) The patient psychogenetically regresses to the oral stage of psychosexual development.

50. *Anhedonia*:
    (a) Is associated with long-term phenobarbitone use.
    (b) Can be detected by a depression rating scale.
    (c) Refers to loss of pleasure in the past.
    (d) Was first described by Anna Freud.
    (e) Is a diagnostic feature of major depression.

PAPER 3

1. *Sick role behaviour*:
   (a) Refers to the effect of unconscious denial.
   (b) Is the activity adopted by those who consider themselves to be ill.
   (c) Refers to the measures taken to prevent disease or detect it in the asymptomatic stage.
   (d) Leads to exemption of normal social obligations.
   (e) Is particularly prolonged in children.

2. *The following statements about premorbid personality are correct*:
   (a) It is reliably assessed by using personality tests.
   (b) One should take into account the last two years of the patient's personality prior to the index illness.
   (c) It should be included in psychodynamic formulation to increase understanding of the presenting problem.
   (d) The patient's own appraisal is adequate.
   (e) It is reliably assessed by the General Health Questionnaire.

3. *The following psychological mechanisms operate in the aetiology of phobic disorders*:
   (a) Preparedness.
   (b) Covert sensitization.
   (c) Learned helplessness.
   (d) Avoidance learning.
   (e) Repression.

4. *The features of sensory distortions include*:
   (a) Change in intensity.
   (b) Tactile hallucination.
   (c) Changes in quality.
   (d) Hyperacusis.
   (e) Changes in spatial form.

5. *Monoamines include*:
   - (a) Glutamate.
   - (b) Dopamine.
   - (c) Glycine.
   - (d) Histamine.
   - (e) GABA (gamma aminobutyric acid).

6. *The following statements about pseudohallucinations are correct*:
   - (a) They are a type of mental image.
   - (b) They are commonly seen in states of clouded consciousness.
   - (c) They are a type of real perceptions.
   - (d) They may occur in dreams.
   - (e) They are located in objective space.

7. *Clinical features helpful in diagnosis of speech disorder in a 40-year-old male include*:
   - (a) Akinesia.
   - (b) Pillrolling tremor.
   - (c) Mid diastolic murmur in the apex.
   - (d) Nystagmus with intention tremor.
   - (e) Painless indolent ulcers in both hands.

8. *The main features of ICD10 (International Classification of Diseases, 10th edition) include the following*:
   - (a) It is produced in a single and elaborate version.
   - (b) F30–F39 refer to mood disorders.
   - (c) The division between neurosis and psychosis is adopted from ICD9.
   - (d) The chapter that deals with mental disorders contains 50 categories.
   - (e) The terms 'neurotic' and 'psychotic' have been excluded from it.

9. *Avoidance conditioning is considered to be involved in the aetiology of*:
   (a) Nocturnal eneuresis.
   (b) Social phobia.
   (c) Obsessional rituals.
   (d) Premature ejaculation.
   (e) Exhibitionism.

10. *Depression of mood may be caused by*:
    (a) Haloperidol.
    (b) Alphamethyldopa.
    (c) Amphetamines.
    (d) Corticosteroids.
    (e) Cimetidine.

11. *Denial is a mechanism commonly seen in*:
    (a) Anorexia nervosa.
    (b) Pathological grief reaction.
    (c) Depression.
    (d) Fugue states.
    (e) Bulimia nervosa.

12. *The serial sevens test*:
    (a) Serves as an indicator of mathematical ability of the patient.
    (b) Is a good indicator of concentration.
    (c) Is a diagnostic test for Alzheimer's disease.
    (d) Is able to differentiate cognitive impairment due to a variety of reasons.
    (e) Is usually impaired in a psychotic patient.

13. *Characteristic features of frontal lobe dysfunction include*:
    (a) Loss of short-term memory.
    (b) Lack of foresight.
    (c) Distractibility.
    (d) Aphasia.
    (e) Depression.

14. *Behavioural assessment of an agoraphobic patient includes:*
    (a) Fear of closed spaces.
    (b) Fear of crowds.
    (c) Recent life events.
    (d) Avoidance of market places.
    (e) Family history.

15. *The common side-effects of tricyclic antidepressant drugs include:*
    (a) Difficulty in micturition.
    (b) Weight gain.
    (c) Excessive sweating.
    (d) Jaundice.
    (e) Prolongation of P–R interval in the electrocardiagraph (ECG).

16. *Prion dementias include:*
    (a) Creutzfeld–Jakob disease.
    (b) Gerstmann–Straussler syndrome.
    (c) Lewy body disease.
    (d) Kuru.
    (e) Krabbe's disease.

17. *Characteristic features of autoscopy include:*
    (a) Visual hallucinations.
    (b) Seeing one's own image.
    (c) Auditory hallucinations.
    (d) Hysterical behaviour.
    (e) Phantom mirror image phenomenon.

18. *A behavioural assessment of phobias will include:*
    (a) Habituation.
    (b) Incubation.
    (c) Preparedness.
    (d) Assimilation.
    (e) Stimulus generalization.

19. *Essential features of post-traumatic syndrome include*:
    (a) Hypervigilance.
    (b) Pervasive anxiety.
    (c) Anhedonia.
    (d) Intolerance to alcohol.
    (e) Exaggerated startle response.

20. *The following statements about muscarinic (M) receptors are correct*:
    (a) M1 receptors are concentrated in the sympathetic ganglia, corpus striatum and stomach.
    (b) They are closely associated with Na^+ channels.
    (c) Pilocarpine is an agonist at muscarinic receptors.
    (d) Dexamethonium and succinylcholine are muscarinic receptor antagonists.
    (e) Muscarinic receptor antagonists have both central and peripheral actions.

21. *Features of borderline personality disorder as described in DSMIIIR include*:
    (a) A pattern of unstable and intense interpersonal relationships characterized by alternation between extremes of over-idealization and devaluations.
    (b) Affective instability.
    (c) Reaction to criticism with feelings of rage, shame or humiliation (even if not expressed).
    (d) Preoccupation with feelings of envy.
    (e) Chronic feelings of emptiness and boredom.

22. *A brain-stem lesion can be distinguished from a cortical lesion by*:
    (a) Blurred vision.
    (b) Dysphagia.
    (c) Vertigo.
    (d) Dysphasia.
    (e) Paralysis of upper limb being worse than that of lower limb.

23. *Flight of ideas characteristically occurs in*:
    (a) Mania.
    (b) Schizophrenia.
    (c) Hypothalamic lesions.
    (d) Schizo-affective disorder.
    (e) Obsessive compulsive disorder.

24. *Potentially fatal interaction occurs by combining a monoamine oxidase inhibitor with*:
    (a) Red wine.
    (b) Caffeine.
    (c) Codeine.
    (d) Propranolol.
    (e) Lithium carbonate.

25. *In analytic psychotherapy, the following are recommended*:
    (a) All the questions must be open-ended.
    (b) The patient is called by his/her first name.
    (c) Eye to eye contact is necessary.
    (d) The therapist should direct the patient.
    (e) Interpretation of dreams and transference.

26. *Nissl substance*:
    (a) Is composed of rough endoplasmic reticulum.
    (b) Appears as coarse granules under a light microscope.
    (c) Synthesizes protein for the nervous system.
    (d) Is a component of lysosomes.
    (e) May be found in the white blood cells.

27. *The following are dosage equivalents of 100 mg of chlorpromazine*:
    (a) Trifluoperazine – 10 mg.
    (b) Droperidol – 4 mg.
    (c) Pimozide – 2 mg.
    (d) Sulpiride – 400 mg.
    (e) Haloperidol – 10 mg.

28. *Characteristic pathological features of vascular dementia include*:
    (a) Pick's bodies.
    (b) Multiple microscopic infarcts.
    (c) Ventricular dilatation.
    (d) Selective asymmetrical atrophy of frontal and temporal lobes.
    (e) Generalized cerebral atrophy.

29. *Characteristic features of perseveration include*:
    (a) Repetition.
    (b) Knight's move.
    (c) Verbal stereotypy.
    (d) Disturbance of the flow of thinking.
    (e) Crowding of thought.

30. *The following support the dopamine hypothesis of schizophrenia*:
    (a) All known effective antipsychotic compounds block dopamine receptors both *in vivo* and *in vitro*.
    (b) Amphetamines in high doses produce a psychosis resembling paranoid schizophrenia.
    (c) Cerebrospinal fluid of schizophrenic patients shows a significant decrease in the metabolism of dopamine.
    (d) Oral administration of dopamine in normal subjects produces a psychosis similar to schizophrenia.
    (e) All the drugs effective in the treatment of schizophrenia invariably raise the prolactin levels.

31. *Tactile hallucinations characteristically occur in*:
    (a) Cocaine psychosis.
    (b) Korsakoff's psychosis.
    (c) Alcoholic hallucinosis.
    (d) Delirium tremens.
    (e) Temporal lobe epilepsy.

32. *The diagnostic criteria of histrionic personality included in ICD10 consist of:*
    (a) Unwillingness to make even reasonable demands on the people one depends on.
    (b) Self-dramatization, theatricality, exaggerated expressions of emotion.
    (c) Suggestibility.
    (d) Limited capacity to make everyday decisions without an excessive amount of advice and reassurance from others.
    (e) Over-concern with physical attractiveness.

33. *Psychoanalytic techniques include:*
    (a) Exploration of parapraxes.
    (b) Repression.
    (c) Hypnosis.
    (d) Free association.
    (e) Interpretation of dreams.

34. *The features of the blood–brain barrier include the following:*
    (a) It separates the blood from the cerebrospinal fluid and the brain.
    (b) Lipid-soluble substances are prevented from entry through the barrier.
    (c) The permeability of the blood–brain barrier to drugs is linked to their water solubility.
    (d) The pH of CSF can be regulated independently of plasma pH.
    (e) Large aminoacids cross the barrier freely.

35. *The past history of the following strongly suggest a diagnosis of schizo-affective disorder:*
    (a) Concomitant treatment with antidepressant and antipsychotic drugs.
    (b) Thought broadcasting.
    (c) Intermingling features of schizophrenia and depression.
    (d) Lithium therapy.
    (e) Intermingling features of schizophrenia and mania.

36. *The following statements about a model psychiatric interview are correct*:
   (a) Start the interview with open-ended questions.
   (b) Mental state examination should be done in a set order.
   (c) Assessment of premorbid personality is highly desirable.
   (d) Occupational and educational history serves as a check on premorbid intelligence.
   (e) Family history helps to understand the dynamics within family members.

37. *Characteristic features of Gerstmann's syndrome include*:
   (a) Finger agnosia.
   (b) Dysphasia.
   (c) Right to left disorientation.
   (d) Dysgraphia.
   (e) Dyslexia.

38. *The symptoms differentiating major depression from anorexia nervosa include*:
   (a) Constipation.
   (b) Loss of weight.
   (c) Anhedonia.
   (d) Low self-esteem.
   (e) Early morning waking.

39. *The mechanisms frequently associated with hysteria include*:
   (a) Identification.
   (b) Sublimation.
   (c) Projection.
   (d) Reaction formation.
   (e) Denial.

40. *The following statements about the cerebral cortex in human beings are correct:*
    (a) The neocortex constitutes about 90% of the cerebral cortex.
    (b) It has six cellular layers.
    (c) It consists of 17 Broadmann's areas.
    (d) It is a sheet of white matter.
    (e) It contains Martinotti cells.

41. *Excessive binge eating occurs in:*
    (a) Thyrotoxicosis.
    (b) Anorexia nervosa.
    (c) Kleine–Levin syndrome.
    (d) Social phobia.
    (e) Grief reaction.

42. *Peripheral effects of anticholinergic drugs include:*
    (a) Pupillary dilation.
    (b) Dry mouth.
    (c) Constriction of bronchi.
    (d) Increased gastric secretions.
    (e) Retention of urine.

43. *Dissociation occurs in:*
    (a) Malingering.
    (b) Automatic writing.
    (c) Twilight state.
    (d) Ganser's syndrome.
    (e) Depersonalization–derealization syndrome.

44. *Little or no activity is seen on EEG record in the following conditions:*
    (a) Multi-infarct dementia.
    (b) Delirium tremens.
    (c) Alzheimer's disease.
    (d) Brain death.
    (e) Huntington's disease.

45. *Characteristic features which differentiate anorexia nervosa from bulimia nervosa include*:
    (a) Body shape disparagement.
    (b) Amenorrhoea.
    (c) Significant weight loss.
    (d) Lanugo hair.
    (e) Selective avoidance of high calorie diet.

46. *Drugs contraindicated in hepatic failure include*:
    (a) Haloperidol.
    (b) Moclobemide.
    (c) Dothiepin.
    (d) Phenelzine.
    (e) Lithium carbonate.

47. *Excessive eating occurs in*:
    (a) Normal weight bulimia.
    (b) Prader–Willi syndrome.
    (c) Diabetes mellitus.
    (d) Major depression.
    (e) Generalized anxiety disorder.

48. *Misidentification*:
    (a) Includes a sense of presence of an identical double.
    (b) Usually occurs in De Clarembault's syndrome.
    (c) Is a normal experience.
    (d) Is a prominent feature of paranoid schizophrenia.
    (e) Is caused by a delusional system.

49. *Components of a neurone include*:
    (a) Neurocyte.
    (b) Nucleus.
    (c) Neuroglia.
    (d) Myelin sheath.
    (e) Synaptic cleft.

50. *The claims of traditional Freudian psychoanalytic theory include the following:*
    (a) The manifest content of dreams refers to the material which the therapist seeks to reveal by means of interpretation.
    (b) The features of secondary process thinking are characteristic of the latent content of dreams.
    (c) The superego represents the fulfilment of ego-ideal.
    (d) 'Dream work' is the patient's effort to reveal the latent content of dreams.
    (e) The 'latency period' causes a resurgence of the sexual drive.

PAPER 4

1. *Learning theories have made a significant contribution in the aetiological understanding of*:
   (a) Agoraphobia.
   (b) Social phobia.
   (c) Obsessive compulsive disorder.
   (d) Fetishism.
   (e) Dissociative states.

2. *Confabulation*:
   (a) Is a characteristic feature of Korsakoff's psychosis.
   (b) Is almost always associated with clouding of consciousness.
   (c) Is due to disorder of temporal sequence of events.
   (d) Is proportional to the degree of anterograde amnesia.
   (e) Is frequently seen in patients suffering from chronic schizophrenia.

3. *The antidepressant action of a psychotropic drug*:
   (a) Is due to blockade of postsynaptic reuptake of 5-hydroxytryptamine.
   (b) Is due to down regulation of beta-adrenergic receptors.
   (c) Is due to blockade of presynaptic reuptake of noradrenaline.
   (d) Is due to blockade of postsynaptic reuptake of dopamine.
   (e) Is due to inhibition of synaptic monoamine oxidases.

4. *The characteristic features of generalized anxiety disorder include*:
   (a) Diplopia.
   (b) Intention tremor.
   (c) Frequent yawning.
   (d) Digital paraesthesia.
   (e) Subjective difficulty in breathing.

5. *Negative automatic thoughts include*:
   (a) Arbitrary abstraction.
   (b) Generalization.
   (c) Selective inference.
   (d) Dichotomous reasoning.
   (e) Categorization.

6. *Denial characteristically occurs in*:
   (a) Bipolar affective disorder.
   (b) Dissocial personality disorder.
   (c) Dissociative states.
   (d) Terminal illness.
   (e) Anorexia nervosa.

7. *The structures involved in pupillary light reflex include*:
   (a) Optic nerve.
   (b) Optic radiation.
   (c) Edinger–Westpal nucleus.
   (d) Occipital cortex.
   (e) Oculomotor nuclei.

8. *Characteristic features which differentiate depression from anorexia nervosa include*:
   (a) Cold peripheries.
   (b) Bradycardia.
   (c) Overactivity.
   (d) Psychomotor retardation.
   (e) Poor appetite.

9. *The following are open-ended questions*:
   (a) What can I do for you?
   (b) Well, it seems that you are in trouble.
   (c) Tell me what is troubling you.
   (d) How are you feeling at the moment?
   (e) So, you are less depressed now?

10. *Most typical symptoms of depression include*:
    (a) Early morning wakening.
    (b) Anhedonia.
    (c) Increased fatigability.
    (d) Diurnal variation in mood.
    (e) Depressed mood.

11. *DSMIIIR contains the following diagnostic categories on Axis I*:
    (a) Neurosis.
    (b) Hysteria.
    (c) Hypochondriasis.
    (d) Schizotypal disorder.
    (e) Late paraphrenia.

12. *The following enhance the passage of psychotropic drugs through the blood–brain barrier*:
    (a) High molecular weight.
    (b) Active metabolite.
    (c) Low protein binding.
    (d) High lipid solubility.
    (e) First bypass.

13. *Depression may be a presenting symptom of*:
    (a) Gastric carcinoma.
    (b) Hypothyroidism.
    (c) Pheochromocytoma.
    (d) Alzheimer's disease.
    (e) Pancreatic carcinoma.

14. *The following statements about pharmacokinetics of chlorpromazine are correct:*
    (a) Its plasma level is increased by concomitant administration of a tricyclic antidepressant drug.
    (b) Its plasma level is decreased by concomitant administration of a selective serotonin reuptake inhibitor drug.
    (c) It reaches a peak concentration level at 3 hours after an oral dose.
    (d) The therapeutic effect is directly proportional to the plasma concentration of the drug.
    (e) Its plasma level is decreased by concomitant administration of an anticholinergic drug.

15. *Recognized features of vitamin B12 deficiency include:*
    (a) Anxiety.
    (b) Depression.
    (c) Paranoid states.
    (d) Delirium.
    (e) Memory impairment.

16. *According to psychodynamic theory:*
    (a) The ego is entirely conscious.
    (b) The id is entirely unconscious.
    (c) The ego operates on secondary process thinking.
    (d) Instinct is inherited and unchangeable.
    (e) The superego is derived from the ego.

17. *Pitfalls in correctly assessing the patient's mood include:*
    (a) Failure to ask about a history of alcohol abuse.
    (b) Failure to ask direct questions.
    (c) Failure to utilize standardized rating scales.
    (d) Inability to recognize the interviewer's own non-verbal behaviour.
    (e) Failure to interact with the patient's non-verbal communication.

18. *Characteristic deficits associated with lesions of*
    non-dominant temporal lobe include:
    (a) Inability to learn new roads.
    (b) Diminution of musical appreciative capacity.
    (c) Difficulty in reproducing visual designs from memory.
    (d) Emotional instability.
    (e) Aggressive behaviour.

19. *The following statements about late paraphrenia are*
    correct:
    (a) Genetic predisposition is considered insignificant.
    (b) The incidence rate is equal in both sexes.
    (c) The patients have a previous history of schizophrenia.
    (d) Sensory deprivation may be important in its aetiology.
    (e) It is an early manifestation of Alzheimer's disease.

20. *The following statements about anticholinesterases are*
    correct:
    (a) They inhibit the enzyme acetyl cholinesterase.
    (b) L-Dopa is an example.
    (c) Physostigmine is an example.
    (d) They may benefit patients suffering from Alzheimer's
        disease.
    (e) They lead to accumulation of acetylcholine at
        cholinergic synapses.

21. *The following drugs possess a major sedative effect in*
    therapeutic dosage:
    (a) Phenelzine.
    (b) Dothiepin.
    (c) Trazodone.
    (d) Fluoxetine.
    (e) Fluvoxamine.

22. *According to psychoanalytic theory of anxiety, the*
    following are important in its aetiology:
    (a) Birth trauma.
    (b) Bereavement.
    (c) Fear of castration.
    (d) Separation.
    (e) Maternal deprivation.

23. *Dendrites*:
   (a) Do not contain mitochondria.
   (b) Are covered by myelin sheath.
   (c) Are found only in the brain.
   (d) Act as synaptic plates.
   (e) Bear spikes which act as sites for synaptic contact.

24. *The following statements about Schneider's first rank symptoms are correct*:
   (a) They are pathognomonic features of schizophrenia.
   (b) They are present in schizophrenic patients across the globe.
   (c) They are not usually found in psychotic patients with mental retardation.
   (d) They are typical of psychosis associated with temporal lobe epilepsy.
   (e) They include Gedankenlautwerden.

25. *Reliability of psychiatric diagnosis*:
   (a) Is improved by operational definitions.
   (b) Is improved by multiaxial classification.
   (c) Does not matter if diagnostic categories have low validity.
   (d) Is improved by semistructured interviews.
   (e) Is no different between unstructured and structured interviews.

26. *The negative symptoms of schizophrenia include*:
   (a) Inappropriate affect.
   (b) Blunted affect.
   (c) Apathy.
   (d) Indifference to the environment.
   (e) Poverty of movement.

27. *Characteristic features of anorexia nervosa include*:
   (a) Loss of pubic hair.
   (b) Loss of at least 25% of body weight.
   (c) Amenorrhoea before significant weight loss.
   (d) Presence of lanugo hair.
   (e) Loss of libido.

28. *Factors that influence the occurrence of sexual dysfunction include*:
    (a) Inadequate information.
    (b) Poor sex education.
    (c) Depression.
    (d) Poor communication.
    (e) Loss of attraction.

29. *Recognized features of narcolepsy include*:
    (a) An association with epilepsy.
    (b) Catalepsy.
    (c) Abnormal electroencephalograph.
    (d) Loss of muscle tone.
    (e) Night terror.

30. *Pseudohallucinations are recognized features of*:
    (a) Borderline syndrome.
    (b) Hypnagogic states.
    (c) Bereavement.
    (d) Fatigue.
    (e) Hypnopompic states.

31. *Characteristic features of Wernicke's encephalopathy include*:
    (a) Nystagmus.
    (b) Ataxia of gait.
    (c) Tremors of the lips.
    (d) Peripheral neuropathy.
    (e) Pernicious anaemia.

32. *According to psychological theories, a simple symptom phobia is due to*:
    (a) Imprinting.
    (b) Learned helplessness.
    (c) Preparedness.
    (d) Incubation.
    (e) Second order conditioning.

33. *In a typical interview schedule, as a first step the interviewer should*:
   (a) Give the patient a proforma to fill in as soon as he or she arrives.
   (b) Ask the patient to give history in his or her own words.
   (c) Ask the patient about his or her main problem.
   (d) Make the patient lie on the couch.
   (e) Give the patient a cursory physical examination.

34. *The hypothalamus*:
   (a) Contains a variety of hormone-secreting cells.
   (b) Receives direct afferent fibres from cerebral cortex.
   (c) Forms the floor of the fourth ventricle.
   (d) Sends major outputs to the pituitary gland.
   (e) Is a part of the diencephalon.

35. *Carl Schneider described the following*:
   (a) Thought echo.
   (b) 'Made' experiences.
   (c) Thought broadcasting.
   (d) Delusional perception.
   (e) 'Second rank' symptoms of schizophrenia.

36. *G-protein-coupled receptors*:
   (a) Are distinct from the effector proteins.
   (b) Have extracellular recognition sites for ligands.
   (c) Link cell surface receptors to a variety of enzymes and ion channels.
   (d) Can increase in number after blocking.
   (e) Effect action only through the adenylcyclase second messenger system.

37. *Carl Jung is associated with the following concepts*:
   (a) Archetypes.
   (b) Dream work.
   (c) Animus.
   (d) Inferiority complex.
   (e) Transitional object.

38. *The patient making the following statements has a first rank symptom of schizophrenia:*
    (a) 'I heard a voice telling me I was going to be killed'.
    (b) 'I know the woman next to me could hear what I was thinking'.
    (c) 'I saw the postman dropping a letter and I knew there was going to be a nuclear war'.
    (d) 'It was a strange force inside my brain that made me break the door'.
    (e) 'I don't seem to be able to think for myself. All my thoughts seem to be my father's'.

39. *The electroencephalograph of a sleeping individual:*
    (a) Shows sleep spindles at the first onset of sleep.
    (b) Can reveal epileptiform discharges which are absent from the waking EEG.
    (c) Typically shows direct entry into REM sleep at the onset of sleep in a patient suffering from epilepsy.
    (d) Shows total sleep time to decrease with advancing age.
    (e) Reveals marked slow activity with K-complexes in stage 3 of sleep.

40. *The selective serotonin reuptake inhibitor drugs include:*
    (a) Citalopram.
    (b) Buspirone.
    (c) Zopiclone.
    (d) Maprotiline.
    (e) Moclobemide.

41. *The following statements about an assessment of suicidal risk are correct:*
    (a) Suicidal intent can vary in severity over a short period of time.
    (b) Asking questions about suicidal ideation increases the risk.
    (c) Denial of the suicide intent implies a relatively high risk.
    (d) Admission of the suicide intent minimizes the eventual risk.
    (e) Previous history of a deliberate self-harm indicates a relatively high risk.

42. *The components of mesolimbic tract include*:
    (a) Red nucleus.
    (b) Substantia nigra.
    (c) Amygdala.
    (d) Caudate nucleus.
    (e) Fornix.

43. *The following statements about obsessional thoughts are correct*:
    (a) They are intrusive and disturbing.
    (b) They are rarely pleasurable.
    (c) They occur in healthy people.
    (d) They are rarely images.
    (e) They are usually acted upon by the patient.

44. *The following drugs possess a major sedative effect in therapeutic dosage*:
    (a) Moclobemide.
    (b) Haloperidol.
    (c) Risperidone.
    (d) Nortriptyline.
    (e) Sertraline.

45. *Carl Jung is associated with the following concepts*:
    (a) Free association.
    (b) Persona.
    (c) Anima.
    (d) Depressive position.
    (e) Character armour.

46. *Characteristic features differentiating pain of psychological origin from pain of physical origin include*:
    (a) Increasing in severity with passage of time.
    (b) Intermittent course.
    (c) Precise anatomical location.
    (d) Relief by placebo.
    (e) Relief by analgesics.

47. *The following statements about interneuronal synapse are correct*:
    (a) All the postsynaptic membranes in human beings are chemosensitive.
    (b) The neuronal transmission at the synapse is in a chemical form.
    (c) Axon-axonic synapses are the anatomical substrates of presynaptic inhibition.
    (d) The synapse acts as a two-way valve for propagation of nerve impulses.
    (e) The subsynaptic membrane is usually thicker than non-synaptic areas of the postsynaptic membrane.

48. *Emotional lability is a characteristic feature of*:
    (a) Delirium tremens.
    (b) Bipolar affective disorder.
    (c) Hysterical personality.
    (d) Alzheimer's disease.
    (e) Simple schizophrenia.

49. *In psychoanalytic terms, anxiety*:
    (a) Diminishes in old age.
    (b) Leads to repression.
    (c) Can be a threat to the superego.
    (d) Can be a warning to the ego.
    (e) Is due to unresolved psychic conflicts.

50. *According to ICD10, the dissociative states include*:
    (a) Somatoform disorders.
    (b) Ganser's syndrome.
    (c) Neurasthenia.
    (d) Multiple personality disorder.
    (e) Hypochondriasis.

PAPER 5

1. *The following adverse effects of lithium carbonate require its immediate discontinuation*:
   (a) Persistent fine tremor.
   (b) Ataxia.
   (c) Slurred speech.
   (d) Persistent polyuria and polydipsia.
   (e) Muscular weakness.

2. *The following statements about in-vivo receptor imaging are correct*:
   (a) Both magnetic resonance imaging and positron emission tomography are useful techniques.
   (b) Affinity of psychotropic drugs to receptors can be accurately calculated.
   (c) It has been shown that clozapine has a much higher affinity at D2 receptors than haloperidol.
   (d) It can be used to provide information on regional localization of receptors.
   (e) Flumazenil is used as a high-affinity ligand for opiate receptors.

3. *Characteristic features of schizophrenic thought disorder include*:
   (a) Pareidolia.
   (b) Omission.
   (c) Clang associations.
   (d) Audible thoughts.
   (e) Derailment.

4. *The following statements about ICD10 are correct*:
   (a) It is developed by the United Nations (UN).
   (b) It is a type of categorical classification.
   (c) It contains only psychiatric disorders.
   (d) It is developed by the American Psychiatric Association.
   (e) The traditional division between neurosis and psychosis is retained.

5. *The following statements about an initial assessment of a psychotic patient are correct:*
   (a) One should confidently confront the psychotic symptoms.
   (b) Colluding with paranoid delusions is a wise step.
   (c) The doctor must be careful to avoid implying any expectations in his questions.
   (d) It is sensible to enquire about psychotic symptomatology first before asking screening questions in other areas.
   (e) Mental state examination may reveal useful information before taking a full history.

6. *The following are intracellular structures in human brain:*
   (a) Neurofibrillary tangles.
   (b) Senile plaques.
   (c) Mitochondria.
   (d) Ependyma.
   (e) Nucleolus.

7. *In behaviour therapy:*
   (a) Operational definitions are used for behaviour patterns.
   (b) Functional analysis of behaviour is an absolute necessity.
   (c) Quantitative rating of behaviour is routinely done.
   (d) Associated cognitions are ignored.
   (e) Schedules of reinforcement are intermittent.

8. *The cognitive theory explanation for panic considers that:*
   (a) The initial attack is a *de novo* event.
   (b) Subsequently avoidance plays a part in maintaining the panic attacks.
   (c) Attacks occur only in response to external stimuli.
   (d) Anxiety attacks in childhood contribute greatly to its occurrence in adult life.
   (e) Bodily sensations are misinterpreted as being indicative of an underlying physical illness.

3

9. *Abnormal voluntary movements typically occur in*:
    (a) Tardive dyskinesia.
    (b) Echopraxia.
    (c) Alzheimer's disease.
    (d) Parkinson's disease.
    (e) Chronic schizophrenia.

10. *The following statements about psychotropic drugs are correct*:
    (a) D2 receptor agonists possess antipsychotic activity.
    (b) Amitriptyline causes dry mouth by antagonism of muscarinic receptors.
    (c) Lorazepam opens chloride channels which enhance GABA transmission.
    (d) Lithium carbonate primarily acts by blocking reuptake of catecholamines.
    (e) Buspirone antagonizes 5HT receptors.

11. *The useful indications for carrying out a CT scan include*:
    (a) Suspicion of a cerebral tumour.
    (b) Suspicion of a subdural haematoma.
    (c) Presence of focal neurological signs.
    (d) Clinical pointers towards a normal pressure hydrocephalus.
    (e) Cerebral oedema.

12. *The following are correctly paired as regards their association*:
    (a) Hysteria – denial.
    (b) Obsession – reaction formation.
    (c) Paranoia – projective identification.
    (d) Bereavement – introjection.
    (e) Depression – turning in on oneself.

13. *The following are known to be of aetiological importance in schizophrenia*:
    (a) Excess of life events prior to the onset of the illness.
    (b) Schizophrenicogenic mother.
    (c) Double-bind communication.
    (d) Decreased dopamine in the mesolimbic system.
    (e) Excess of perinatal complications.

14. *The following statements about the blood–brain barrier are correct*:
    (a) It bypasses hepatic metabolism.
    (b) It ultimately depends on the permeability of the capillary membrane.
    (c) It mainly occurs at cerebellar tentorial level.
    (d) It is a selectively permeable system.
    (e) It is guided by 'pH partition hypothesis'.

15. *The operational criteria for the diagnosis of schizophrenia include*:
    (a) DSMIV.
    (b) Schneider's first rank symptoms.
    (c) ICD10.
    (d) Bleuler's fundamental and accessory symptoms.
    (e) Research diagnostic criteria.

16. *Abrupt withdrawal of tricyclic antidepressant drugs may be followed by*:
    (a) Relapse of depression.
    (b) Nausea.
    (c) Vomiting.
    (d) Anxiety.
    (e) Convulsions.

17. *Ruminations*:
    (a) Are characteristically distressing.
    (b) Are usually associated with rituals.
    (c) Are often resisted and not acted upon.
    (d) Are considered a prodromal symptom of schizophrenia.
    (e) Are a normal experience.

18. *The electroencephalogram pattern*:
    (a) Significantly alters with hypnosis.
    (b) Usually does not change with maturation after age of 10 years.
    (c) Is characteristically altered by serotonin reuptake inhibitor drugs.
    (d) Remains abnormal for at least 3 months following a first course of electroconvulsive therapy.
    (e) In a newborn full-term baby is characterized by a relative absence of electrical activity.

19. *Sublimation*:
    (a) Is prominent in conversion hysteria.
    (b) Is associated with fixation at oral stage.
    (c) Is a neurotic ego defence mechanism.
    (d) Involves diversion of immediate gratification to something else.
    (e) Means diversion of unacceptable impulses to acceptable outlets.

20. *Patients with a fear of blushing*:
    (a) Usually avoid well-lit rooms.
    (b) Often suffer from social phobia.
    (c) Are more vulnerable when bored.
    (d) Would often feign toothache.
    (e) Often abuse alcohol.

21. *The following statements about an initial interview of a patient who abuses alcohol are correct*:
    (a) The family members should not be involved at this stage.
    (b) Therapeutic goals should be set at the outset.
    (c) Enquiries should be made about trouble with police.
    (d) The CAGE questionnaire should be applied to identify at-risk drinkers.
    (e) Enquiry about the time of the first drink of the day is not important.

22. *The hypothalamic structures include*:
    (a) Suprachiasmatic nucleus.
    (b) Premamillary nucleus.
    (c) Red nucleus.
    (d) Paraventricular nucleus.
    (e) Olive nucleus.

23. *The recognized features of motor neurone disease include*:
    (a) Amnesia.
    (b) Dysarthria.
    (c) Dysphagia.
    (d) Intention tremor.
    (e) Uncontrollable laughter.

24. *Lack of selective attention is implicated in behaviour patterns occurring in*:
    (a) Dissociative states.
    (b) Alzheimer's disease.
    (c) Depression.
    (d) Schizophrenia.
    (e) Anorexia nervosa.

25. *Lesions in the following structures are associated with significant memory loss*:
    (a) Caudate nucleus.
    (b) Substantia innominata.
    (c) Anterior nucleus of the thalamus.
    (d) Hypothalamus.
    (e) Globus pallidus.

26. *The following are disorders of form of speech*:
    (a) Perseveration.
    (b) Pressure of speech.
    (c) Psychomotor retardation.
    (d) Confabulation.
    (e) Flight of ideas.

27. *Normal experiences include*:
    (a) Near-death experiences.
    (b) Pseudohallucinations.
    (c) Ideas of reference.
    (d) Panoramic memory.
    (e) Delusional mood.

28. *A neurotoxic reaction is characterized by*:
    (a) Ataxia.
    (b) Nystagmus.
    (c) Hyporeflexia.
    (d) Psychomotor retardation.
    (e) Extensor plantar response.

29. *In dynamic psychopathology, 'epinosic gain'*:
    (a) Is usually secondary to intrapsychic conflicts.
    (b) Results in control of anxiety.
    (c) May result in control over people important to the patient.
    (d) Is a simultaneous expression of drives and defences.
    (e) Assists the maintenance of symptoms.

30. *The following statements about an electroencephalograph (EEG) are correct*:
    (a) Alpha rhythm is most prominent over the occipital lobe.
    (b) Low frequency and high amplitude activity is predominantly noticed in waking adults.
    (c) Alpha rhythm is attenuated by the opening of eyes.
    (d) It exhibits desynchronization in the superficial layers of the cerebral cortex.
    (e) Normal EEG rhythms do not vary after the age of 20 years.

31. *Abnormal perceptions include*:
    (a) Auditory hallucination.
    (b) Gustatory hallucination.
    (c) Complex visual hallucination.
    (d) Hypnagogic hallucination.
    (e) Hypnopompic hallucination.

32. *Receptors*:
    (a) Have recognition sites that occur on the neuronal cell body.
    (b) Have a life span up to 6 months.
    (c) Are synthesized in the synapses.
    (d) Can be labelled in post-mortem brain tissue.
    (e) Can have their synthesis altered by certain drugs.

33. *Typical dissociative states include*:
    (a) Catalepsy.
    (b) Somnambulism.
    (c) Night terrors.
    (d) Cataplexy.
    (e) Hysterical amnesia.

34. *In dynamic psychopathology, working alliance*:
    (a) Is based on childhood relationships that have enabled the patient to develop basic trust.
    (b) Is a neurotic, irrational but reasonable rapport between the therapist and the patient.
    (c) Enables the patient to undergo psychoanalysis despite the transference impulses.
    (d) Makes it possible for the patient to achieve an insight.
    (e) Refers to countertransference relationship with the patient.

35. *The components of the blood–brain barrier include*:
    (a) Arachnoid membrane.
    (b) Endothelial lining of the brain capillaries.
    (c) Myelin sheath.
    (d) Gliovascular membrane.
    (e) Capillary basement.

36. *Blood supply of the internal capsule is provided by*:
    (a) Anterior cerebral artery.
    (b) Middle cerebral artery.
    (c) Posterior cerebral artery.
    (d) Anterior choroidal artery.
    (e) Internal carotid artery.

37. *The recognized unwanted effects of antimuscarinic drugs include*:
    (a) Euphoria.
    (b) Dry mouth.
    (c) Insomnia.
    (d) Constipation.
    (e) Drowsiness.

38. *In psychodynamic concepts, the term 'schizoid' means*:
    (a) Brief psychosis.
    (b) Unable to verbalize feelings.
    (c) Being detached, aloof and humourless.
    (d) Diffuse identity.
    (e) Splitting of the self.

39. *Typical features of schizoid personality include*:
    (a) Withdrawal from social contacts.
    (b) Avoidance of competitive situations.
    (c) Intemperate outbursts of anger.
    (d) A tendency to distort friendly actions of others as hostile.
    (e) Tenacious sense of personal rights.

40. *Spasmodic torticollis in a 30- to 50-year-old*:
    (a) Is almost always psychogenic in origin.
    (b) Responds to behaviour therapy.
    (c) May be a presenting symptom of Parkinson's disease.
    (d) May require surgical correction.
    (e) Is certainly psychogenic if the patient can abolish it
        temporarily by touching the face on the same side.

41. *A functional behavioural analysis*:
    (a) Uses a subjective account by the patient of antecedents
        of the problem.
    (b) Uses the assumption that immediate consequences are
        the key determinant of behaviour.
    (c) Includes an operational definition of the behaviour.
    (d) Aims to define the problem and identify key variables.
    (e) Consists of a highly detailed account of predisposing
        factors.

42. *The processes involved in the maintenance of bulimia nervosa include*:
    (a) Overconcern about shape and weight.
    (b) Binges that are maintained by the continued dieting.
    (c) Purgative and diuretic misuse.
    (d) The undermining of the patient's self-control and self-esteem.
    (e) Marked depression.

43. *Placebo-effect in clinical drug trials refers to*:
    (a) The tendency to react to the shape and size of the drug preparation.
    (b) The tendency to improve on the basis of expectancy and mental attitude even to dummy preparations.
    (c) A superficial and short-lived response to active drug preparation.
    (d) The tendency to respond to the colour of drug presentation.
    (e) Worsening of a patient's condition in the placebo group.

44. *The following statements about DSMIV are correct*:
    (a) It is an atheoretical classification.
    (b) It does not contain the word 'neurosis'.
    (c) It uses operational criteria.
    (d) It retains two kinds of hierarchy of psychiatric classification.
    (e) It is a typical example of multiaxial classification.

45. *Brain structures involved in the corneal reflex include*:
    (a) Oculomotor nerve.
    (b) Optic radiation.
    (c) Trigeminal nerve.
    (d) Facial nerve.
    (e) Spinal nucleus of the trigeminal nerve.

46. *The relative merits of categorical classification include the following*:
    (a) It makes it easy to describe the psychiatric disorders.
    (b) The disorders which lie halfway between two disorders are given special attention.
    (c) It is a more flexible system than dimensional classification.
    (d) It is based on aetiological factors.
    (e) It does not strain the resources of a conservative and largely innumerate profession.

47. *Structures involved in pupillary reaction include*:
    (a) Retina.
    (b) Median forebrain bundle.
    (c) Optic tracts.
    (d) Ciliary ganglion.
    (e) Pupillary sphincter.

48. *The ego*:
    (a) Is responsible for the interests of the person as a whole.
    (b) Is in a dependent relation to the claims of the id.
    (c) Is a concept used by Kleinian analysts.
    (d) Is the expression of the defensive pole of the personality in neurotic conflict.
    (e) Is reality oriented.

49. *The following statements about psychiatric history-taking are correct*:
    (a) Sometimes the general history should be taken after the mental state examination.
    (b) During the first few minutes the patient should be allowed to talk freely about whatever he or she wants.
    (c) Direct questions should never be asked.
    (d) The interview should begin by explaining the exact purpose of the interview.
    (e) Non-verbal clues are as important as verbal clues.

50. *Capgras' syndrome is*:
   (a) Allied to hysteria.
   (b) Also called pure erotomania.
   (c) Allied to free association.
   (d) Characterized by delusions of double.
   (e) Is usually associated with paranoid schizophrenia.

PAPER 6

1. *With regard to obsessions*:
T (a) They are sometimes difficult to distinguish from delusions.
T (b) They are always recognized by the subject as being their own thoughts. Obsession cannot be.
F (c) The pathognomonic feature is resistance. ego alien
F (d) In some cases they can be pleasurable.
T (e) They may present as 'magical thinking'.

2. *The following statements about the auditory pathway are correct*:
(a) It sends efferents to the superior temporal gyrus.
(b) The sensory receptors are in the organ of Corti.
(c) Damage to the internal capsule can cause unilateral deafness.
(d) Unilateral lesions of Heschl's gyrus are accompanied by unilateral deafness.
(e) Low frequency sounds are relayed in the superior olivary complex.

3. *The following tests and the areas of the brain tested are correctly matched*:
T (a) Wisconsin card sorting test – frontal lobe.
T (b) Wecshler Adult Intelligence Scale – temporal lobe.
F (c) Grasp reflex – parietal lobe.
T (d) Benton visual retention test – occipital lobe.
F (e) Testing for apraxias – frontal lobe.

4. *Symptoms suggestive of an aura of complex partial seizures include*:

T (a) Forced thinking.

F (b) Nausea.

T (c) Vomiting.

T (d) Abdominal pain.

F (e) Delusional mood.

5. *Projective identification*:

F (a) Is equivalent to empathy.

F (b) Is the same as projection.

T (c) Is a characteristic defence mechanism associated with paranoid–schizoid position.

F (d) Is equivalent to countertransference.

T (e) Is a primitive ego defence mechanism.

6. *Reliability of diagnosis in psychiatric disorders*:

F (a) Is high for schizophrenia with the use of Bleuler's criteria.

T (b) Is improved, along with validity, with the use of operational criteria. → only improve reliability

F (c) Is generally high for psychiatric disorders because the criteria are polythetic.

F (d) Is high for histrionic personality disorder.

T (e) Is high for antisocial personality disorder.

7. *Alcoholic hallucinosis*:

T (a) Can present with visual hallucinations.

F (b) Is more common in those with withdrawal seizures.

T (c) Can lead to persecutory delusions.

T (d) Can be distinguished from delirium tremens on the basis of intact consciousness alone.

F (e) Occurs only after complete discontinuation of drinking.

8. *The neuronal membrane*:
   (a) Resists the passage of ions during its resting state.
   (b) Maintains the potential difference across its membrane through ion pumps.
   (c) Has ion channels for three major ions, Na^+, K^+ and Cl^-.
   (d) Has separate channels for ions that move in and those that move out.
   (e) Depolarizes with increased negativity of the transmembrane potential.

9. *In somatization disorder, the following are considered to be of aetiological importance*:
   T (a) Heightened awareness of bodily sensations.
   F (b) Childhood sexual abuse.
   T (c) History of family illness during childhood.
   F (d) Excessive anxious preoccupation with illness.
   T (e) Misinterpretations of normal sensations as evidence of illness.

10. *In information processing, selective attention involves*:
    T (a) Filtering.
    T (b) Concentrating.
    T (c) Pigeonholing.
    F (d) Telescoping.
    T (e) Categorizing.

11. *The following are correctly paired associations*:
    F (a) Seligman – agoraphobia.
    T (b) Freud – free association.
    T (c) Melanie Klein – paranoid/schizoid position.
    T (d) Donald Klein – panic.
    F (e) Kraepelin – hypnosis.

12. *Non-sedating antidepressants include*:
    T (a) Citalopram.
    T (b) Moclobemide.
    T (c) Sertraline.
    T (d) Paroxetine.
    T (e) Fluoxetine

13. *In the cerebral cortex*:
    (a) The paleocortex contains five layers.
    (b) The neocortex has six layers.
    (c) The neocortex has five basic types of neurones.
    (d) The limbic system is a part of the paleocortex.
    (e) The horizontal cells of Cajal form the innermost layer of the neocortex.

14. *A diagnosis of depression is compatible with the presence of*:
    T (a) Obsessions.
    T (b) First rank symptoms.
    F (c) Elated mood.
    T (d) Past history of schizophrenia.
    T (e) Alcohol dependence.

15. *The following neuropathological findings and conditions are correctly matched*:
    T (a) Status spongiosus – prion dementia.
    T (b) Atrophy of the head of caudate nucleus and putamen – Huntington's disease.
    F (c) Petechial haemorrhages in the mamillary bodies – herpes simplex encephalitis.
    T (d) Hirano bodies – Pick's disease.
    F (e) Lewy bodies – dementia of frontal lobe type.

16. *With regard to the association areas of the cerebral cortex*:
    (a) They are divided into primary and secondary association areas.
    (b) The secondary areas have more widespread projections.
    (c) They receive input from the relay nuclei of the thalamus.
    (d) They perform an integrative function.
    (e) They form a much larger proportion of the cortex in comparison to the primary motor and sensory cortex.

17. *Salient features that differentiate ICD10 schizophrenia from DSMIIIR schizophrenia include*:
    F (a) A lack of classification for the course of schizophrenia.
    T (b) Absence of the subtype simple schizophrenia.
    T (c) A longer duration of psychotic symptoms required to diagnose schizophrenia.
    T (d) Exclusion of first rank symptoms from the criteria.
    F (e) A specified duration for the presence of prodromal symptoms.

18. *Variables adversely affecting the outcome of grief reaction include:*
    T (a) Overdependence on the lost person.
    T (b) Losses that are socially stigmatizing.
    F (c) Poor prior physical health.
    T (d) Loss which occurs in circumstances where the survivor can be blamed.
    T (e) Lack of social support.

19. *Medical students' interviewing skills can be improved by*:
    F (a) Giving a detailed handout.
    T (b) Watching someone experienced interviewing.
    T (c) Using structured interview schedules.
    T (d) Videotape feedback.
    F (e) Psychodrama groups.

20. *Ego strength*:
    T (a) Is an important prerequisite for psychoanalytic therapy.
    T (b) Is found to be very high amongst highly successful people.
    T (c) Includes an ability to integrate interpretations.
    F (d) Is developed during the anal stage.
    F (e) Includes an ability to replace reality with fantasy.

21. *In mania*:
  F (a) The diagnosis can only be made in the presence of elated mood.
  F (b) Grandiose delusions are specific to mania.
  F (c) Decreased attention span suggests an alteration of consciousness.
  T (d) A decreased need for sleep is a useful early warning sign.
  F (e) Psychotic features like delusions and hallucinations are more common than in depression.

22. *Alexithymia*:
  F (a) Is classified under somatoform disorders in the DSMIIIR.
  T (b) Is measured by Beck's depression rating scale.
  F (c) Refers to people who can describe feelings they do not experience.
  F (d) Is usually seen in individuals who are imaginative.
     (e) Is a personality type in which individuals concentrate
  F on their subjective experiences rather than external events.

23. *Side-effects of tricyclic antidepressants that mimic depressive symptoms include*:
  T (a) Tachycardia.
  T (b) Dry mouth.
  F (c) Blurred vision.
  T (d) Postural hypotension.
  T (e) Black tongue.

24. *Each of the following features can reliably distinguish mania from schizophrenia*:
  T (a) Elated mood.
  T (b) Grandiose delusions.
  F (c) Acute onset.
  T (d) Absence of auditory hallucinations.
  T (e) Sexually disinhibited behaviour.

25. *In operant conditioning:*

F (a) When a rat is given a shock in one end of a box and runs to the other end, the learning process is called 'avoidance training'.

F (b) When a rat presses a lever more often because it obtains food, it is called 'survival training'.

F (c) If the rat responds by running away at the sound of a bell, rung before a shock is delivered, this is called 'escape training'.

(d) If the rat is given a shock with no way of escape or avoidance it is called 'punitive training'.

(e) When a rat is given gradually increasing levels of current, it is called 'habitual training'.

26. *The following statements about involuntary movements are correct:*

F (a) In cerebellar disease tremors occur at rest.

T (b) Parkinsonian tremor has a rate of 4–7 cycles per second.

T (c) Fasciculations indicate disease of the lower motor neurone.

F (d) Dyskinesias persist during sleep.

F (e) Meige's syndrome is the eponymous label for blepharospasm.

27. *The following are neuroleptic drugs:*

T (a) Loxapine.

T (b) Pericyazine.

F (c) Carbamazepine.

T (d) Fluspiriline.

T (e) Prochlorperazine.

28. *A 45-year-old man is brought to the Accident and Emergency department in an acutely disturbed state. The diagnosis of a functional psychosis as opposed to an organic psychosis is suspected if he exhibits:*

F (a) Microscopic visual hallucinations.

T (b) Derogatory auditory hallucinations.

(c) Delusions of grandeur.

F (d) Disinhibited behaviour.

F (e) Amnesia for recent events.

29. *The following statements are true about cognitive testing in the elderly*:
   (a) The CAMDEX is part of a larger battery of tests, the CAMCOG.
   (b) The Mini Mental State is helpful in distinguishing dementia from pseudodementia.
   (c) Most tests contain assessment for aphasia.
   (d) Cognitive deficits can even be diagnosed by the MMPI.
   (e) The Hatchinski scale is used to diagnose multi-infarct dementia.

30. *In psychoanalytic theory, ego functions include*:
   (a) Mediation between the id and the outside world.
   (b) Resolution of sexual conflict.
   (c) Reality testing.
   (d) Defensive functions.
   (e) Object relationships.

31. *The ion channels in the neuronal membrane*:
   (a) Are responsible for the action potential.
   (b) Are only electrically activated.
   (c) Are selective for the type of ion to which they are permeable.
   (d) Are only chemically activated.
   (e) Open when the depolarization reaches the spike threshold.

32. *The negative symptoms of schizophrenia include:*
   (a) Thought blocking.
   (b) Incongruous affect.
   (c) Avolition.
   (d) Confabulation.
   (e) Psychomotor retardation.

33. *Spatial disorientation is a recognized feature of:*
   (a) Puerperal psychosis.
   (b) Korsakoff's psychosis.
   (c) Alcoholic hallucinosis.
   (d) Alzheimer's disease.
   (e) Ganser's syndrome.

34. *The following statements about life events are correct*:
  (a) Suicide attempters report more events than depressives.
  (b) In contrast to other psychiatric disorders, depression occurs specifically following interpersonal loss.
  (c) Endogenous depression is more likely to be related to life events.
  (d) Different types of life events occur in depressed as compared to anxious patients.
  (e) The risk of developing depression continues to increase with time, after the event.

35. *Neuropathological features that are found in patients with AIDS include*:
  (a) Cerebral atrophy.
  (b) Thickening of the meninges.
  (c) Spongy degeneration of the white matter tracts.
  (d) Lacunar infarcts.
  (e) Diffuse astrocytosis.

36. *Features described as prodromal symptoms of schizophrenia in the ICD10 include*:
  (a) Loss of interest in work.
  (b) Generalized anxiety.
  (c) Marked depression.
  (d) Auditory hallucinations.
  (e) Poor personal hygiene.

37. *Autoscopy*:
  (a) Is a primary delusion.
  (b) Is a type of depersonalization experience.
  (c) Is compatible with normality.
  (d) Is a characteristic feature of right parietal/occipital infarct.
  (e) Is the same as doppelgänger.

38. *Evoked potentials*:
   F (a) Are recorded while stimuli from multiple sensory
        modalities are presented to the subject.
   T (b) Require the background electrical activity to be
        averaged out.
   F (c) Include the P300, which is an early potential.
   T (d) Have been shown to be consistently abnormal in type 2
        schizophrenia.
   T (e) Classified as late potentials, reflect cognitive processing.

39. *Postulated psychodynamic factors in the aetiology of
    anxiety disorders include*:
   T (a) Homosexual libidinal drives.
   T (b) Threatened emergence into consciousness of forbidden
        repressed psychic conflicts.
   T (c) Fear of castration.
   T (d) Response to external threat.
   F (e) Breaking off of affectional bonds.

40. *Normal persons may experience the following*:
   T (a) Depersonalization.
   T (b) Hypnagogic hallucinations.
   T (c) *Déjà vu*.
   T (d) Irrational fear of harmless objects.
   T (e) Disorientation in time, place and person.

41. *Termination of the neurotransmitter effects in a
    serotonergic synapse is influenced by*:
   F (a) Reuptake into the postsynaptic membrane.
   T (b) Monoamine oxidases.
   T (c) Genomic factors.
   T (d) Diffusion.
   T (e) Receptor adaptation.

42. *In functional behavioural analysis:*
  (a) A history of the patient's social relationships is irrelevant.
  (b) Clarification of the circumstances that maintain a problem behaviour forms an important component.
  (c) The defence mechanisms responsible for the problem behaviour are analysed.
  (d) The frequency and intensity of major complaints including hallucinations are analysed.
  (e) Motivational analysis is included.

43. *The following are components of the extended cognitive state examination:*
  (a) Comprehensive evaluation of language functions.
  (b) Level of conscious awareness.
  (c) Evaluation for dyspraxia.
  (d) Visuospatial and constructional difficulties.
  (e) Evaluation for formal thought disorder.

44. *Circumstantiality:*
  (a) Is a disorder of stream of thoughts.
  (b) Has been described as approximate answers in Ganser's syndrome.
  (c) Is synonymous with tangentiality.
  (d) Is a characteristic feature in schizophrenia.
  (e) Occurs in people with learning disability.

45. *With regard to the neuronal excitation:*
  (a) The resting potential is normally negative inside.
  (b) Closing of the Na$^+$ channels results in the accumulation of the positive ions.
  (c) The action potential lasts from 1 to 2 ms.
  (d) After an action potential the neurone is temporarily less excitable.
  (e) Hyperpolarization occurs as the Na$^+$ ions move out of the cell.

46. *The following paired terms are equivalent in their meanings*:
- F (a) Pressure of speech – flight of ideas.
- T (b) Blunted affect – affective flattening.
- F (c) Dysphoria – anhedonia.
- T (d) 'Made' action – delusion of control.
- F (e) Perseveration – confabulation.

47. *The transitional object, as described in dynamic psychopathology*:
- F (a) Is replaced by the permanent object as the child grows older.
- F (b) Was first described by Melanie Klien.
- T (c) Represents a substitute for the mother's breast.
- F (d) Is an important component of the Oedipal stage of psychosexual development.
- T (e) Is usually a favourite toy.

48. *A patient being treated with a reversible inhibitor of monoamine oxidase A, should not partake of*:
- F (a) Pickled herrings.
- F (b) Aged cheese.
- F (c) Cottage cheese.
- F (d) Red wine.
- F (e) Yeast products.

49. *Observational learning*:
- T (a) Is an important form of learning in childhood.
- T (b) Includes 'modelling'.
- T (c) Is an effective treatment for phobias.
- F (d) Is a part of 'respondent learning'.
- T (e) Requires a behavioural sequence and its consequences to be observed.

50. *The following are the basic classes of second messengers*:
- T (a) Cyclic nucleotides.
- F (b) Monoamines.
- T (c) Calcium ions.
- F (d) RNA.
- T (e) Phospholipid metabolites.

$\dfrac{178}{220} = 80.90\%$

ANSWERS TO PAPER 1

1. (a) T. Neuritic or senile plaques are extracellular argyrophilic bodies which also occur in normal elderly people.
   (b) T.
   (c) T. These are small eosinophilic neuronal inclusion bodies.
   (d) F. They are a part of the cortical pathology of dementia associated with Parkinson's disease.
   (e) T. It is a deposition of amyloid around small blood vessels. Alzheimer's disease type 2 is an early onset dementia, i.e. before the age of 65.

2. (a) F. Catatonia also occurs in organic and affective disorders.
   (b) F.
   (c) T. In *Mitmachen*, the body can be put into any position without any resistance on the part of the patient, even though he or she has been instructed to resist all movements.
   (d) F. *Gedankelautwerden* is a German name for audible thoughts which describes the patient's experience of hearing his own thoughts said out loud. Its French version is *echo de la pensées*.
   (e) F. It was first introduced by Karl Kahlbaum. Kasanin described schizo-affective psychosis.

3. (a) F.
   (b) F.
   (c) T.
   (d) T.
   (e) T.

4. (a) F. 'Paranosic' means primary advantage derived from an illness, i.e. primary gain. Item (a) refers to a secondary gain.
   (b) T.
   (c) T.
   (d) F. It refers to secondary gain.
   (e) T.

5. (a) T.
   (b) T.
   (c) F. Risperidone is an antagonist at the central serotonergic S2 receptors.
   (d) F. It is an antagonist at both the noradrenergic and histaminergic receptors.
   (e) F.

6. (a) T.
   (b) T. It is one of the most striking features. The person is rigid in his or her views and inflexible in his or her approach to problems.
   (c) T. As in (b).
   (d) T. It is one of the most striking features. The person finds it hard to weigh up the advantages and disadvantages of new situations.
   (e) F. This is a feature of antisocial/dissocial personality disorder.

7. (a) T. This is a special method of psychotherapy invented by Freud, dealing particularly with transference.
   (b) F. Dynamic psychotherapy is concerned with the largely unconsciously derived and transferred feelings and attitudes with which the patient invests in the analyst.
   (c) T.
   (d) F.
   (e) T. It includes analysis of unconscious conflicts, deficits and distortions of intrapsychic structures and internal object relations.

8. (a) T. Although the mental state examination is largely concerned with what the patient says, much can also be learned from observing his or her general appearance, behaviour, mood, posture and movement.
   (b) T.
   (c) F. This indicates the patient's subjective feelings.
   (d) T.
   (e) T.

9. (a) T.
   (b) T.
   (c) F. It decreases beta (high frequency) activity and increases delta and/or theta (low frequency) activity.
   (d) F. It increases delta (low frequency) activity.
   (e) F. It produces insignificant EEG changes.

10. (a) T.
    (b) F.
    (c) T.
    (d) F.
    (e) F. Being identical twins *per se* is not associated with increased incidence of schizophrenia. However, if one of the twins develops schizophrenia, the other twin has a much higher incidence rate than the general population.

11. (a) F. Obsessive compulsive disorder characteristically uses regression, intellectualization and other defence mechanisms as mentioned in (b), (d) and (e).
    (b) T.
    (c) F.
    (d) T.
    (e) T.

12. (a) T. The id is a completely unconscious intrapsychic
        agency that is only interested in discharging tension.
   (b) T. The conscious aspect of the ego is the executive
        organ of the psyche, responsible for decision making
        and integration of perceptual data. The unconscious
        aspect of the ego contains the defence mechanisms.
   (c) T.
   (d) T. For most part the superego is unconscious, but
        aspects of it are certainly conscious. The conscious
        level of functioning involves 'secondary processes'
        which are logical, rational and geared to meet the
        demands of the real world.
   (e) T.

13. (a) T. The overriding effect of damage to the upper motor
        neurones is a withdrawal of inhibition from spinal
        reflexes, resulting in hyperreflexia and hypertonia.
   (b) T. Wernicke's aphasia is a disorder of reception which
        leads to impairment of comprehension of spoken
        language.
   (c) T.
   (d) T. When the superficial plantar reflex is abolished by
        upper motor neurone lesion, Babinski's sign is
        unmasked.
   (e) F.

14. (a) F. The amount excreted in breast milk is too small to
        be harmful.
   (b) T. A significant amount of sulpiride is excreted in
        milk.
   (c) F. As in (a).
   (d) T.
   (e) F. As in (a).

15. (a) T.
   (b) F. Visual hallucinations usually occur in organic
        brain disorders or psychotic disorders.
   (c) T.
   (d) F.
   (e) T.

16. (a) F. The EEG changes consist of intermittent diffuse irregular delta (low frequency) activity which increases after each treatment. EEG returns to normal within 3 months of the treatment.
    (b) T.
    (c) F. The plasma cortisol levels are raised after a single treatment and the rise lasts for 2 to 4 hours.
    (d) T. Changes in blood pressure mirror changes in pulse rate.
    (e) F. The cerebral circulation increases dramatically during either spontaneous or electrically induced epileptic seizures. ECT seems to produce a large increase in the blood–brain barrier permeability.

17. (a) T.
    (b) F. The aetiology of Wilson's disease is known but it is not classified as a psychiatric disorder.
    (c) T.
    (d) F. The aetiology of Alzheimer's disease is unknown.
    (e) F. The aetiology of Briquet's syndrome is unknown.

18. (a) F. The central feature of this syndrome is a loss or impairment of function which appears to be due to a physical cause but is in fact a manifestation of some underlying psychological conflict or need. The symptoms reduce unconscious anxiety.
    (b) F.
    (c) F. The hysterical conversion symptoms are mediated via the peripheral nervous system.
    (d) T.
    (e) F. The conversion symptoms usually confer some advantage on the patient by producing primary and secondary gains.

19. (a) T.
    (b) F. This area is associated with expressive speech.
        The lesions lead to expressive dysphasia.
    (c) T. The other structures associated with memory include
        amygdala, uncus and dorso-medial nucleus of the
        thalamus.
    (d) T.
    (e) F.

20. (a) T. Posterior columns (medial leminiscal pathways)
        convey conscious and discriminative touch.
    (b) F.
    (c) T.
    (d) T. They provide the parietal lobe with an instantaneous
        body image, so that we are constantly aware of the
        body parts both at rest and during movements.
    (e) F.

21. (a) T. The id represents all the inherited, biological and
        constitutional features of the individual including
        instincts and basic drives.
    (b) F. The ego is reality oriented and finds acceptable and
        appropriate ways of satisfying the demands of the id
        and superego.
    (c) T. As in (e).
    (d) T.
    (e) F. The id operates according to the hedonistic pleasure
        principle in that it avoids being frustrated and seeks
        immediate gratification, regardless of the
        consequences.

22. (a) F. Dopamine release promotes drive reinforcement and
        an experience of pleasure.
    (b) T.
    (c) F.
    (d) F. Depletion of dopamine leads to Parkinson's disease
        and possibly other movement disorders.
    (e) T.

23. (a) F. Return to work is unusual and complete recovery is rare. Improvement tends not to occur after the financial settlement.
    (b) T.
    (c) T.
    (d) F. These patients may have some difficulty with sleep.
    (e) F. The central feature is the seeking of financial compensation after sustaining a relatively trivial injury.

24. (a) F. In reflection, although a part of what the patient says is repeated, it is not necessarily an exact repetition of what the patient says.
    (b) F. Direct questions are used to gather specific information.
    (c) F. The answer to item (c) is clarification.
    (d) F. Silence is a very important component of interviewing.
    (e) F. Recapitulation, i.e. summation, would be logical only at the end of the interview.

25. (a) T. Haptic or tactile hallucinations may be experienced as sensations of being touched, pricked or strangled.
    (b) T.
    (c) F.
    (d) F. Hallucinations of bodily sensation are common in schizophrenia, cocaine addition and alcohol withdrawal.
    (e) T.

26. (a) F. Most diagnoses are dependent on multiple symptoms rather than single symptoms.
    (b) T.
    (c) T.
    (d) F. There are few validating criteria such as laboratory tests.
    (e) F. When inferences need to be drawn as in determining psychodynamic defence mechanisms, the reliability tends to be poor.

27. (a) F. Graded hierarchies are used where the patient grades all the situations avoided in order of difficulty.
    (b) F. For maximum effectiveness exposure should be graduated, repeated and prolonged and the interval between the sessions should be short.
    (c) F. As in (b).
    (d) T. As in (b).
    (e) F. As in (b).

28. (a) T.
    (b) F.
    (c) T.
    (d) T.
    (e) F.
    Papilloedema (optic disc swelling due to raised intracranial pressure) is usually bilateral and produces enlargement of the blind spot without loss of acuity. The causes of papilloedema include posterior uveitis, posterior scleritis, optic neuritis, anterior ischaemic optic neuropathy, optic nerve sheath meningioma, sarcoidosis, leukaemia and lymphoma.

29. (a) F. Atropine poisoning is characterized by dry mouth, blurred vision, difficulty in swallowing, dilated pupils, flushed skin, tachycardia, delirium and myoclonus.
    (b) T.
    (c) T.
    (d) T.
    (e) F. Hallucinogenic type mushroom (*Psilocybe* and *Panaeolus* species) poisoning is characterized by mydriasis, nausea, vomiting and intense visual hallucinations.

30. (a) F.
    (b) T.
    (c) F.
    (d) T.
    (e) T.
    Dothiepin, trazodone and benztropine possess anticholinergic action which results in dryness of mouth, constipation, difficulty in micturition and blurred vision.

31. (a) F. Purkinje cell axons are only efferent fibres from the cerebellar cortex which travel to other parts of the brain.
    (b) F. Like the climbing fibres – the terminal fibres of olivocerebellar tracts, mossy fibres are the terminal fibres of all other cerebellar afferent tracts. They do not send direct innervation to the Purkinje cells.
    (c) T. The inhibitory signals from the Purkinje cells contribute to the final output from the cerebellum.
    (d) T. Pathologically, hereditary ataxia of Pierre-Marie is indistinguishable from other hereditary degenerations or Friedreich's ataxia.
    (e) T. Other efferents are to the vestibular and reticular neurones and the thalamus.

32. (a) F. Eidetic imagery is an intense and detailed visual image. It is an experience within the mind, usually without the sense of reality that is part of perception.
    (b) F.
    (c) T.
    (d) F.
    (e) T. It is usually obliterated by seeing or hearing.

33. (a) T.
    (b) T.
    (c) F.
    (d) T.
    (e) T.
    Changing the topic (switching) or explaining away things as if they are expected (normalization) as well as improper reassurance frequently lead to inadequate information being obtained.

34. (a) T.
    (b) F. Transference is not interpreted in supportive psychotherapy.
    (c) F. Transference is not a response to countertransference or vice versa. Countertransference is the analyst's own strong feeling toward a patient.
    (d) T.
    (e) T.

35. (a) T. The major pathological changes in Alzheimer's
             disease include widespread cerebral atrophy,
             neuronal loss, neuritic plaques and neurofibrillary
             tangles.
    (b) T.
    (c) F. See (d).
    (d) F. Histological changes include cortical neuronal loss
             and neurofibrillary degeneration with neurofibrillary
             tangles in the cortex and brain stem. Neuritic
             plaques, however, are not present.
    (e) T. They are a core of paired helical filaments of
         F   uncertain nature.

36. (a) T. Normal grief is characterized by three stages.
             The first stage is characterized by a lack of emotional
             reaction ('numbness') and a feeling of unreality that
             lasts from a few hours to several days. In the second
             stage, the person feels sad, weeps, sleeps badly and
             loses appetite. In the third stage, these symptoms
             subside gradually and the person accepts the new
             situation.
    (b) F.
    (c) F.
    (d) T.
    (e) T.

37. (a) F.
    (b) T.
    (c) T.
    (d) T.
    (e) T.

38 (a) F. Primacy is given to thoughts and attitudes
(cognitions).
  (b) T. Ellis' rational emotive therapy was influential in the
development of cognitive behaviour therapy.
  (c) T. A schema is a particular set of attitudes and beliefs
through which the individual appraises and
interprets his or her environment, other people and
him/herself.
  (d) F. The depressive triad is Beck's concept.
  (e) F. Events tend to activate negative ways of thinking and
precipitate depression in vulnerable persons.

39. (a) F.
    (b) F.
    (c) F.
    (d) F.
    (e) F.
Reciting the months of the year in reverse order is a test of
concentration.

40. (a) T. About half of the patients have episodes of
uncontrollable overeating during which they may
eat large amounts of food that is usually avoided.
    (b) F.
    (c) F.
    (d) T. Bulimia refers to episodes of uncontrolled excessive
eating.
    (e) T. Some depressed patients eat more and gain weight.
It seems that eating brings temporary relief to their
distressing feelings.

41. (a) F. It may be associated with anorexia and with weight
loss.
    (b) F. It produces gastrointestinal disturbances,
constipation and anorexia.
    (c) F.
    (d) F.
    (e) T.

42. (a) T. Schedules of reinforcement refer to the pattern or
frequency with which a reinforcer is delivered as a
consequence of behaviour.
 (b) F. As in (a).
 (c) F. As in (a).
 (d) T.
 (e) T.
Variable interval schedule is another type of reinforcement
schedule.

43. (a) T.
 (b) F.
 (c) T.
 (d) T.
 (e) T.
In brief focal dynamic psychotherapy, 5 to 20 sessions
might be allocated depending on the complexity of the
problems. The therapist emphasizes that the patient will be
helped to find his of her own solutions to the problems.

44. (a) T. Acetylcholine is the primary excitatory transmitter at
the neuromuscular junction and preganglionic
autonomic nerves.
 (b) F.
 (c) T See (a).
 (d) F. Dopamine is the principal neurotransmitter involved
with the mesolimbic tract.
 (e) T. See (a).
There are two distinct types of acetylcholine receptors:
the nicotinic which gate a sodium channel and the
muscarinic which are linked to the G protein and
phosphoinositol cycle.

45. (a) T. Cognitive events refer to conscious, identifiable
thoughts and images present in the stream of
consciousness.
 (b) F.
 (c) F.
 (d) T. Cognitive processes refer to the processing of
information.
 (e) T. Cognitive structures refer to attitudes or beliefs.

46. (a) T.
    (b) F. It is a sign of anorexia nervosa.
    (c) F. As in (b).
    (d) T.
    (e) T.

47. (a) T.
    (b) T.
    (c) T.
    (d) T.
    (e) T.

48. (a) F. Alcohol abuse is under the same grouping as abuse of other drugs.
    (b) F. All mood disorders have been brought under the same grouping, as opposed to ICD9 in which depression occurred in 13 different categories.
    (c) F.
    (d) T.
    (e) F. ICD9 was not produced after field trials.

49. (a) T. The early clinical feature is one of dissociated sensory loss.
    (b) T.
    (c) F. Sensitivity to touch is retained because the posterior column is preserved.
    (d) T. Patients develop ulcers on the fingers arising from painless cuts and burns.
    (e) F.

50. (a) T.
    (b) T. They are often associated with sleepwalking.
    (c) T.
    (d) F. Night terrors occur in stages 3 and 4 of sleep which are associated with low frequency delta and theta rhythm. Alpha rhythm is between 8 Hz and 13 Hz.
    (e) F. As in (d).

ANSWERS TO PAPER 2

1. (a) F. Post-psychotic depression is included under schizophrenia.
   (b) T.
   (c) T.
   (d) F.
   (e) F. Neither narcissistic nor passive aggressive personality disorder has been included in ICD10.

2. (a) T.
   (b) T.
   (c) F.
   (d) T.
   (e) F.

3. (a) T. Due to variability in responding that occurs with fixed schedules, variable schedules are used to get smooth patterns of responding.
   (b) T.
   (c) T.
   (d) T. 'Scalloping' refers to the increase in responding that occurs as the time for reinforcement draws nearer.
   (e) T.

4. (a) F.
   (b) T.
   (c) F.
   (d) T.
   (e) F.

5. (a) T. Bell's palsy is a common disorder caused by a neuritis (possibly viral in origin) of the facial nerve. Facial paralysis is usually complete on the affected side.
   (b) T. The patient is unable to raise the eyebrow, close the eye or retract the lip.
   (c) T.
   (d) T.
   (e) F.

6. (a) F. It indicates a long-term memory.
   (b) F. It indicates the level of concentration.
   (c) T.
   (d) T.
   (e) F. It indicates a long-term memory.

7. (a) T.
   (b) F.
   (c) T.
   (d) T.
   (e) T.

8. (a) T.
   (b) T.
   (c) T. The tongue is contracted and spastic and cannot be moved rapidly from side to side.
   (d) T.
   (e) F. The patient experiences difficulty in swallowing, chewing, coughing, breathing and talking (dysarthria).

9. (a) T.
   (b) T.
   (c) F.
   (d) T.
   (e) T.
   Depersonalization and derealization are experienced quite commonly as transient phenomena by healthy adults and children, especially when tired. The experience usually begins abruptly and in normal people seldom lasts more than a few minutes. The symptoms may occur after sleep deprivation.

10. (a) T.
    (b) F. They have three intracellular loops.
    (c) F. They have an extracellular N-terminal.
    (d) F. They have an intracellular C-terminal.
    (e) F. The G-protein receptors form one of the superfamilies of central nervous system receptors; a superfamily consists of receptors that share several common features.

11. (a) F. In the cognitive model, it is not the events *per se* but
      people's expectations and interpretations that are
      responsible for negative emotions.
    (b) T. As in (a).
    (c) F. Perceived loss is important in depression.
    (d) T.
    (e) F. The patient's responses are considered inappropriate
      and out of proportion to the perceived danger.

12. (a) T. Classically there is an asymmetry with reduced
      amplitude activity on the affected side, but more
      often there is an increased localized irregular slow
      activity with sharp waves.
    (b) F.
    (c) F.
    (d) T. The typical finding is of generalized, widespread
      slow (theta) wave activity occurring in 31% to 58%
      of psychopaths. The 'positive-spike' phenomenon is
      found in 40% to 45% of aggressive and impulsive
      psychopaths.
    (e) T. Here extremely slow focal delta waves are recorded.

13. (a) T. Supportive psychotherapy is used to help a person
      through a time-limited crisis caused by either social
      problems or by physical illness.
    (b) T.
    (c) F. It is an essential part of analytic psychotherapy.
    (d) F. As in (c).
    (e) T. Other important features include listening,
      explanation, reassurance, prestige suggestion.

14. (a) F. There is a multiaxial presentation in Chapter V (F)
      of ICD10 but it is not used in the main classification.
    (b) F. ICD10 covers psychiatric disorders occurring in all
      age groups.
    (c) T.
    (d) F. ICD10 refers to the word 'hysteria' in the chapter on
      neurotic, stress-related and somatoform disorders
      (F40 to F48). However, the hysterical disorders are
      referred to as dissociative conversion disorders.
    (e) F. Only Chapter V CF refers to psychiatric disorders.

15. (a) F.
    (b) T.
    (c) F.
    (d) F.
    (e) F.
The main principles of the diagnostic interview include the following:
    (1) Start by giving the patient free rein to describe his or her problems as he or she sees them.
    (2) Symptoms which are complained of spontaneously are always more convincing than those elicited only by direct questioning.
    (3) The initial questions on any topic should always be as wide and open-ended as possible.
    (4) Never ask questions in such a way that you make it clear which answer you are expecting.
    (5) Record the patient's replies to key questions and any striking or unusual remarks verbatim.

16. (a) T.
    (b) F.
    (c) T.
    (d) F.
    (e) T.

17. (a) F. There is a generalized atrophy of the cerebral cortex with widening of the sulci and enlargement of the ventricular systems.
    (b) T. As in (a).
    (c) T. It is the most striking feature of Alzheimer's disease.
    (d) F. Acetylcholine neurones are mainly affected.
    (e) T.

18. (a) T.
    (b) F.
    (c) T.
    (d) T.
    (e) T. Other common side-effects include dry mouth, sedation, blurred vision, sweating.

19. (a) F. It descends through the corona radiata and the internal capsule and passes through the ventral part of the mid brain, medulla oblongata and travels down the spinal cord.

(b) F. The pyramidal or crossed motor (lateral cortico-spinal) tracts unlike the direct or uncrossed motor (anterior corticospinal) tracts decussate in the medulla oblongata and then pass inferiorly to the opposite side of the spinal cord.

(c) T. The degeneration of pyramidal tracts leads to ataxia with a wide-based and stamping gait, loss of vibration and deep pain sensation and a positive Romberg's sign.

(d) F. This high speed and large diameter system connects the cerebral cortex to the ventral horns of the spinal cord, without intervening synapses.

(e) F. It terminates mainly on interneurones in the dorsal horns of the spinal cord and a small portion directly on the anterior motor neurones. Renshaw cells are inhibitory interneurones in the anterior horn of the spinal cord.

20. (a) T. Hypomanic patients are overactive and restless.

(b) T.

(c) F.

(d) F. Anxious patients are often tremulous and restless.

(e) T. Akathisia is an unpleasant feeling of physical restlessness and a need to move, leading to an inability to keep still.

21. (a) T.
    (b) F. Histological changes include neuronal loss in the cerebral cortex particularly affecting the frontal lobes and in the corpus striatum, particularly affecting GABA neurones.
    (c) F. A characteristic histological feature is the presence of argyrophilic intracytoplasmic neuronal inclusion bodies known as Pick's bodies, consisting of neurofilaments, paired helical filaments and endoplasmic reticulum.
    (d) T. There are multiple cerebral infarcts and local or general atrophy of the brain with secondary ventricular dilatation.
    (e) F. Other conditions associated with neurofibrillary tangles include postencephalitic Parkinsonism, the Parkinsonism-dementia complex of Guam, amyotrophic lateral sclerosis, progressive supranuclear palsy, also patients who have received aluminium through renal dialysis.

22. (a) T.
    (b) T.
    (c) T.
    (d) F.
    (e) T. Depersonalization is particularly associated with generalized and phobic anxiety disorders, depressive disorders, schizophrenia and sensory deprivation.

23. (a) F. In normal males, REM sleep is invariably associated with a penile erection.
    (b) T. This is associated with loss of libido.
    (c) F. Penile erection is generally unimpaired but generalized anxiety disorder may be associated with loss of libido and premature ejaculation.
    (d) F.
    (e) T. The exact mechanism of penile erection is not completely understood. It is a consequence of stimulation of sacral parasympathetic fibres or sympathetic inhibition which triggers the vascular response.

24. (a) F. The main defence mechanism employed in phobias is displacement, whereas conversion is the main defence mechanism with conversion disorder.
    (b) T.
    (c) F. In both these disorders, the defence mechanisms involved are the same, i.e. repression, displacement and avoidance.
    (d) T.
    (e) F. Isolation and undoing are the defence mechanisms important for obsessive compulsive disorders and not social phobia.

25. (a) T.
    (b) T.
    (c) T.
    (d) T.
    (e) T.
    Other common side-effects include nausea, tremor, insomnia, agitation and increased sweating.

26. (a) T.
    (b) F. The id, ego and superego are a structural model of the mind.
    (c) F. Freud described Oedipal complex in boys and Electra complex in girls.
    (d) T.
    (e) T.

27. (a) T.
    (b) T.
    (c) F.
    (d) T.
    (e) T.
    Psychiatric disorders presenting physical symptoms are heterogeneous and difficult to classify. It is probable that most symptoms arise in part from the misinterpretation of normal bodily sensations and trivial physical complaints, distress being expressed in bodily rather than psychological terms.

28. (a) F. These receptors form one of the superfamilies of brain receptors.
    (b) T. Ionotropic receptors also include nicotinic cholinergic receptors, GABA-A receptors and kainate receptors.
    (c) T.
    (d) T.
    (e) T. Because of the rapid changes of neuronal excitability that occur when these receptors are stimulated, the drugs acting on these receptors have a narrow therapeutic window.

29. (a) T.
    (b) T.
    (c) T.
    (d) F. It is a primitive defence mechanism.
    (e) F. As in (d).

30. (a) T.
    (b) F. It is a part of the archiocortex.
    (c) F. It is a part of the paleocortex.
    (d) T.
    (e) T.

    From a developmental point of view, the cerebral cortex consists of three parts:
    (1) the paleocortex;
    (2) the archicortex;
    (3) the neocortex, i.e. new structures.

    The neocortex becomes prominent in mammals and it achieves its greatest development in primates. In human beings, it constitutes about 90% of the cerebral cortex.

31. (a) T.
    (b) F. Serial sevens is a test of concentration and not short-term memory.
    (c) T.
    (d) F.
    (e) F. Three repetitions of such a sentence are usually enough for correct immediate reproduction by a healthy young person. However, this test does not satisfactorily discriminate patients with organic brain disorder from patients with depressive disorder or even from healthy young people.

32. (a) T.
    (b) T.
    (c) T.
    (d) T.
    (e) F. The EEG pattern of REM sleep is similar to that of stage 1 of non-REM sleep, i.e. low frequency theta activity, with superimposed sawtooth waves. Within the sleeping time, the proportion of REM sleep to non-REM sleep diminishes from approximately 50% in the new-born full-term baby to less than 20% by middle age.

33. (a) F. Amnesia may occur on recovery. The patients are likely to show memory disturbance and disorientation while having clouded consciousness.
    (b) T.
    (c) F. Clouding of consciousness denotes the mildest stage of impairment of consciousness on a continuum from full alertness and awareness to coma.
    (d) T.
    (e) T.

34. (a) F. It is characterized by motor restlessness, a subjective feeling of tension and an inability to tolerate inactivity which gives rise to restless movement. Acute akathisia occurs in some 20% of patients receiving antipsychotic drugs and comes on within the first few weeks of treatment.
    (b) T.
    (c) F. Tardive dyskinesia is more common among women, the elderly and patients who have diffuse brain pathology. In half of the cases, it appears when the drugs are stopped.
    (d) F. Acute dystonia occurs in 2% to 10% of patients treated with antipsychotic drugs.
    (e) T. Routine administration of such drugs is not justified as not all patients are affected and because tardive dyskinesia may be unmasked or worsened by them. These drugs are abused for their mood-altering effects.

35. (a) F. Self-psychology is derived from the seminal writings of Heinz Kohut. It stresses how external relationships maintain self-esteem and self-cohesion.
    (b) T.
    (c) T.
    (d) F. It is of particular help while treating narcissistic patients.
    (e) F. Object relations theory is derived from the work of Melanie Klein, Fairburn, Winnicott and Balint.

36. (a) T.
    (b) T.
    (c) T.
    (d) T.
    (e) F. Parietal lobe syndrome is characterized by visuo-spatial difficulties such as constructional apraxia and visuo-spatial agnosia, topographical disorientation, visual inattention, sensory Jacksonian fits and cortical sensory loss.

37. (a) T. Echolalia means that the patient refers to words or parts of sentences that are spoken to him/her or in his/her presence.
  (b) F. Cataplexy refers to sudden temporary episodes of paralysis with loss of muscle tone. It is one of the characteristic features of narcolepsy.
  (c) T. Psychological pillow refers to a condition in which the patient's head is maintained a few inches above the bed for a sustained period which may continue for hours.
  (d) T. Stereotypy refers to a bizarre uncomfortable posture which may be retained for some hours.
  (e) T. Echopraxia refers to a symptom in which the patient imitates the interviewer's every action.

38. (a) F. Object relations theory differs from ego psychology in two important ways:
    (i) It considers drives as secondary and not primary.
    (ii) It has compressed the development time-table of classical theory into the first year of life.
  (b) T.
  (c) T.
  (d) F. D.W. Winnicott coined the phrase 'good enough mothering'.
  (e) T.

39. (a) T. The experience of the passage of time is also well known to vary in different, normal circumstances. When the person is happy or engrossed, the time seems to pass very fast; when sad, bored or idle, time drags.
  (b) T.
  (c) T.
  (d) T.
  (e) T.

40. (a) F. The two-step conditioning process was hypothesized to underlie the development of fear and by analogy, the phobic disorder.
  (b) F.
  (c) F. The first step involves the pairing of a stimulus situation with fear (classical conditioning).
  (d) T.
  (e) T. The second step involves reinforcing avoidance of the now feared situation by anxiety reduction (operant conditioning).

41. (a) T. ICD10 is designed to be a central ('core') classification for a family of disease- and health-related classifications. Chapter V refers to mental and behavioural disorders.
  (b) T.
  (c) F. Distinguishing between different grades of severity remains a problem. In mood disorders, three grades of mild, moderate and severe forms of disorders have been specified. There is a separate coding for somatic, psychotic or mixed symptoms in certain diagnostic categories.
  (d) F. ICD10 is considered suitable for both primary health care and hospital care.
  (e) T.

42. (a) T.
  (b) T.
  (c) T.
  (d) T.
  (e) T. Other features include vertical furrows on the brow, hunched shoulders with sitting leaning forward.

43. (a) F.
  (b) F. Punch-drunk syndrome is characterized by cerebellar, pyramidal and extrapyramidal signs as well as intellectual deterioration.
  (c) T.
  (d) F. The most frequent symptoms include muscular atrophy and spasticity with exaggeration of tendon reflexes.
  (e) F.

44. (a) T.
    (b) F.
    (c) F.
    (d) T.
    (e) F. Differentiation from hypochondriacal delusions usually depends upon close acquaintance with the patient. Although the beliefs are long-standing and appear to be held against reason, the degree of conviction is usually susceptible.

45. (a) F.
    (b) F.
    (c) T.
    (d) T.
    (e) F. It is a phenomenon observed in group psychotherapy where some patients may become 'scapegoated' because of their more primitive psychopathology and their greater tendency to express affect in a direct manner.

46. (a) T.
    (b) T. The skeletal muscles are innervated by nerves which originate in the lower motor neurones of the anterior grey column and in the motor nuclei of the cranial nerves.
    (c) T. This leads to flaccid paralysis, hypotonia, decreased deep tendon reflexes and muscle wasting in poliomyelitis.
    (d) F.
    (e) F. In this infection, i.e. herpes zoster, the cells of the posterior root ganglion are affected leading to eruptions of vesicles and change of colour of the skin in the affected area.

47. (a) T.
    (b) T.
    (c) F. Learned helplessness is not a symptom of depression.
    (d) T.
    (e) F.
    In 1975, Seligman suggested that depression developed when reward or punishment is no longer clearly contingent on the actions of the organism.

48. (a) F.
    (b) F.
    (c) F. The dosage should be reduced.
    (d) F. As in (c).
    (e) T.

49. (a) T.
    (b) T.
    (c) F. Bibring believed that depression was a primary affective state unrelated to aggression turned inwards.
    (d) T. In psychoanalytic understanding, depression is similar to melancholia and mourning. Freud suggested that the causes of mourning and depression might be similar, e.g. mourning results from loss by death and depression results from actual loss or a loss of 'some abstraction'.
    (e) T.

50. (a) T.
    (b) T.
    (c) T.
    (d) F.
    (e) T.

Anhedonia means total inability to enjoy anything in life or even get the accustomed satisfaction from usual leisure activities.

ANSWERS TO PAPER 3

1. (a) F. Sick role behaviour was first described by Talcott Parsons in 1951. It does not involve any judgement by the doctor as to whether the processes involved are conscious or unconscious.
   (b) T.
   (c) F.
   (d) T. The other right of the sick individual is exemption from blame for the illness.
   (e) T.
   Parsons described two obligations: (1) a wish to recover and (2) to accept the appropriate help.

2. (a) F. Aspects of a patient's premorbid personality can be judged by asking him/her for his/her own self-rating, by asking other people who know him/her well, and by observing his/her behaviour at interview.
   (b) F. Good indications of premorbid personality can often be obtained by asking the patient or others how he/she has behaved in particular circumstances.
   (c) T.
   (d) T. The patient's own account of his/her premorbid personality may be distorted by his/her illness or a general lack of insight.
   (e) F. The General Health Questionnaire (GHQ) is a self-rated 60 item questionnaire designed to identify psychiatric 'cases'. It was designed for use in a community setting, primary care or general medical out-patients.

3. (a) T. Preparedness is an inherited biological trait and a concept used in learning theory.
   (b) F. It is the use of aversive stimuli in imagination in the management of deviant sexual behaviours and urges.
   (c) F. Seligman suggested that depression develops when reward or punishment is no longer clearly contingent on the action of the organism.
   (d) T.
   (e) T. The source of anxiety is excluded from consciousness by repression and attached to the manifest object by displacement.
   A reasonable suggestion is that phobic symptoms are due to a combination of conditioning and abnormal cognitions (fear of evaluation).

4. (a) T. In sensory distortions there is a constant real perceptual object which is perceived in a distorted way such as changes in intensity, quality and spatial form.
   (b) F. It is a type of sensory deception which occurs without an adequate external stimulus.
   (c) T. As in (a).
   (d) T. Here the threshold at which sound is perceived as unpleasantly loud is lowered, i.e. there is a generalized increase in sensory input.
   (e) T. As in (a).

5. (a) F. It is an aminoacid.
   (b) T. Other monoamines include noradrenaline, adrenaline and serotonin.
   (c) F. As in (a).
   (d) T.
   (e) F. As in (a).

6. (a) T. Although the mental image is clear and vivid, it lacks the substantiality of perceptions.
   (b) F. They are seen in full consciousness and are known to be not real perceptions.
   (c) F. As in (b).
   (d) F. Dreams occur in rapid eye movement (paradoxical) sleep. Pseudohallucination is perhaps the most likely phenomenological form to describe the apocalyptic experience of visions.
   (e) F. They are always located in subjective space and perceived with the inner eye or ear.

7. (a) T.
   (b) T. The patient with postencephalitic Parkinson's disease speaks slowly and articulates poorly, slurring over many syllables and trailing off the end of sentences. The voice is low-pitched, monotonous and lacks inflection.
   (c) F.
   (d) T. In cerebellar lesions, the principal speech abnormality is slowness; imprecise enunciation, monotony and unnatural separation of the syllables of the words.
   (e) T. Syringobulbia which never occurs without syringomyelia may extend into the lateral tegmentum of the medulla. Unilateral paralysis of the palate and vocal cords as well as weakness and atrophy of one side of the tongue occur.

8. (a) F. ICD10 is available in several different versions.
   (b) T.
   (c) F. The terms 'neurosis' and 'psychosis' are not adopted; however, 'neurotic' and 'psychotic' are used in descriptive terms.
   (d) F. The chapter that deals with mental disorders has 100 categories.
   (e) F. As in (c).

9. (a) F.
   (b) T.
   (c) T. Avoidance of objects or situations which trigger
       obsessions is one of the core features of obsessional
       problems.
   (d) F.
   (e) F.
   The avoidance of or relief from distressing emotion is
   frequently an immediate effect of a problem behaviour and
   is often the most potent maintaining factor.

10. (a) T.
    (b) T.
    (c) F. They produce euphoria.
    (d) T.
    (e) F. It is not associated with depression or elevation of
        mood.

11. (a) T.
    (b) T.
    (c) T.
    (d) T.
    (e) T.
    Denial is a direct disavowal of traumatic sensory data.
    It is ordinarily a defence against the external world of
    reality when that reality is overwhelmingly disturbing.
    Although it is associated primarily with psychoses and
    severe personality disorders, it may also be used by normal
    people, especially in the face of catastrophic events.

12. (a) F. Serial sevens is a test of attention and concentration.
    (b) T.
    (c) F. It is grossly impaired in Alzheimer's disease, but not
        as such a diagnostic test.
    (d) F. Performance depends on educational and intellectual
        attainment and arithmetic skills.
    (e) F. It may be impaired in psychotic patients.

13. (a) T.
    (b) T. It is a failure to anticipate the consequence of a
           course of action.
    (c) T.
    (d) F.
    (e) F.

14. (a) T.
    (b) T.
    (c) F.
    (d) T.
    (e) F.
    Behavioural assessment consists of a highly detailed
    account of the current determinants of the agoraphobic
    problem rather than its historical antecedents, predisposing
    or precipitating factors.

15. (a) T.
    (b) T.
    (c) T.
    (d) F.
    (e) F. The common change in ECG is a prolongation of the
           Q–T interval.

16. (a) T. Prion dementias, i.e. subacute spongiform
           encephalopathy, are characterized by the
           accumulation in the brain of an abnormal form of a
           normal host protease-resistant protein, PrP, hence the
           name 'prion'.
    (b) T. It is inherited as an autosomal dominant gene with
           complete penetrance.
    (c) F. Lewy bodies are eosinophilic intracellular inclusions
           which are present in the basal ganglia and substantia
           nigra of patients with Parkinson's disease.
    (d) T.
    (e) F. Also known as globoid cell leuko-dystrophy or
           galactosylceramide lipidosis. It is caused by a
           deficiency of the enzyme galacto-cerebroside-B-
           galactosidase, which leads to an accumulation of
           galacto-cerebroside in the central and peripheral
           nervous systems.

17. (a) T. It is the experience of seeing oneself and knowing that it is oneself. It may take the form of a pseudohallucination.
    (b) T. As in (a).
    (c) F. It may involve several modalities of sensation; but auditory hallucination is not a characteristic feature.
    (d) F. Autoscopy is occasionally described as a hysterical behaviour.
    (e) T. Phantom mirror image and autoscopy are synonymous.

18. (a) F. Habituation is based on the idea that the practical task early in training is repeated and predictably used to elicit thoughts over the period required for anxiety reduction, while at the same time preventing any covert avoidance and neutralizing behaviours.
    (b) F.
    (c) T. The theory of 'preparedness' applies to phobias of small animals, illness, or injury, thunderstorms, heights, strangers and water, and to situations such as being far away from a safe place and being rejected by other people. It means that the things feared may be or have been potentially dangerous to the human race.
    (d) F.
    (e) T. Stimulus generalization occurs when a response which has been conditioned to one stimulus is produced by another stimulus without any additional learning having taken place.
    Behavioural assessment of phobias includes phobic severity, maintaining factors, existing coping skills and graded hierarchies.

19. (a) T.
    (b) T.
    (c) T.
    (d) F. Excessive use of alcohol or drugs may be a complicating factor.
    (e) T.

20 (a) T.
   (b) F. They are closely associated with K$^+$ channels and are regulated by gallamine, GTP and inhibit adenyl cyclase.
   (c) T.
   (d) F. They are, in fact, nicotinic receptor antagonists.
   (e) T. They include confusion, lassitude and drowsiness, and dry mouth, excessive sweating, blurring of vision and urinary retention respectively.

21. (a) T.
    (b) T.
    (c) F. A diagnostic feature of narcissistic personality disorder.
    (d) F. As in (c).
    (e) T.

22. (a) F. The causes of blurred vision vary with age. They include myopia, presbyopia, cataracts, glaucoma, retinal haemorrhages and detachments.
    (b) T.
    (c) T. Vertigo of brain-stem origin implicates vestibular nuclei and their connections. In these cases auditory function is nearly always spared. There are attendant signs of involvement of cranial nerves, sensory and motor traits etc., and nystagmus.
    (d) T. It may also occur in cortical lesions.
    (e) F.

23. (a) T. Flight of ideas is an acceleration of the flow of thinking in which there is no general direction and the connection between successive thoughts appears to be due to chance factors.
    (b) F. It occasionally occurs in excited schizophrenic patients.
    (c) T. As in (a).
    (d) T. As in (a).
    (e) F.

24. (a) T. Alcohol containing tyramine interacts with MAO inhibitors and produces hypertensive crisis.
    (b) F. Caffeine is a weak stimulant present in tea and coffee. It is included in many analgesic preparations but does not contribute to their analgesic or anti-inflammatory effect.
    (c) T. MAOI and opioid analgesics interactions include CNS excitement or depression (hypertension or hypotension).
    (d) F.
    (e) F.

25. (a) F. The psychiatrist must maintain a flexible interviewing style that shifts from a structured pursuit of specific facts (e.g. symptoms, family history, life events, duration of illness) to an unstructured posture of listening to the natural ebb and flow of the patient's thought processes.
    (b) F. It is a good practice to call the patient by his/her first name but only with the patient's permission.
    (c) F.
    (d) F. The therapist must simply create an atmosphere in which the patient feels free to talk. He or she can learn a great deal by allowing the patient to ramble freely for a while.
    (e) T. Interpretations are made about the patient's behaviour within or outside the therapeutic sessions (such as acting out countertransference, parapraxes, unconscious conflict, deficits and distortions of intrapsychic structures).

26. (a) T. The Nissl substance (chromophil substance) is the most characteristic of nerve cells.
    (b) T.
    (c) T.
    (d) F. Lysosomes are spherical membrane-surrounded bodies containing a number of powerful enzymes and act as the neuronal digestive system or as internal scavengers.
    (e) F. As in (a).

27. (a) F. The correct dosage equivalent is 5 mg.
    (b) T.
    (c) T.
    (d) F. The correct dosage equivalent is 200 mg.
    (e) F. The correct dosage equivalent is 3 mg.

28. (a) F. They are characteristic of Pick's disease.
    (b) T. They may also be macroscopic infarcts.
    (c) T.
    (d) F. This is a characteristic feature of Pick's disease.
    (e) T.

29. (a) T. In perseveration – a disorder of the continuity of thinking – a word, phrase or idea persists beyond the point at which it is relevant.
    (b) F. Knight's move or derailment refers to a transition from one topic to another, either between sentences or in mid sentence, with no logical relationship between the two topics.
    (c) F. Here the same word or phrase is used regardless of situation.
    (d) T. As in (a).
    (e) F. Here the patient describes his thoughts as being passively concentrated and compressed in his head. The associations are experienced as being excessive in amount and outside the patient's control.

30. (a) T.
    (b) T.
    (c) F. There is no convincing evidence as to identifying an increase in metabolites of dopamine in the cerebrospinal fluid (CSF) of schizophrenic patients.
    (d) F. Oral dopamine is absorbed in the gastrointestinal tract.
    (e) T.

31. (a) T. Tactile hallucinations, sometimes called haptic hallucinations, are experienced as sensations of being touched, pricked or strangled. They may also be felt as movements just below the skin which the patient may attribute to insects, worms or other small creatures burrowing through tissues.
    (b) F.
    (c) F.
    (d) T. As in (a).
    (e) F. Hallucinations of smell, taste, vision, hearing or bodily sensations, and distorted perceptions occur in temporal lobe epilepsy.

32. (a) F. A diagnostic feature of dependent personality disorder.
    (b) T.
    (c) T.
    (d) F. As in (a).
    (e) T.

33. (a) T.
    (b) F. It is an ego defence mechanism which operates unconsciously by expelling unacceptable wishes, feelings or fantasies from conscious awareness.
    (c) F. Hypnosis has been used in a variety of conditions such as control of pain and anxiety.
    (d) T.
    (e) T.

34. (a) T.
    (b) F. Lipid-soluble substances pass readily through the barrier.
    (c) F. As in (b).
    (d) T. The pH of CSF can be regulated independently of plasma pH, because un-ionized CO_2 passes across the barrier much more readily than bicarbonate ions.
    (e) T.

35. (a) F.
    (b) T. ?F
    (c) T.
    (d) T.
    (e) T.
    Schizo-affective disorder is an episodic disorder in which
    both affective and schizophrenia symptoms are prominent
    within the same episode of illness, preferably simultaneously,
    but at least within a few days of each other. Such patients
    usually respond to ECT, neuroleptics and lithium
    carbonate, but not often to tricyclic antidepressant drugs.

36. (a) T.
    (b) T.
    (c) T.
    (d) T.
    (e) T.
    The psychiatric interview serves as a psychiatrist's main
    tool of investigation. It is a technique of obtaining
    information and serves as a standard situation in which to
    assess the patient's emotions and attitudes.

37. (a) T. Gerstmann's syndrome is a particular form of body
           image disturbance resulting from a dominant
           parietal lobe lesion; other features include acalculia
           and colour agnosia. The condition may occur in the
           absence of any other form of body image
           disturbance.
    (b) F.
    (c) F. ? T
    (d) T.
    (e) F.

38. (a) F.
    (b) F. Most patients suffering from major depression do
        not have a desire for excessive weight loss or
        excessive fear of gaining weight, whereas in anorexia
        nervosa the weight loss should be at least 15% of
        normal body weight.
    (c) T.
    (d) F. Depressed mood and lability of mood are common
        features of anorexia nervosa. In chronic cases,
        hopelessness and thoughts of suicide may be present.
    (e) F.

39. (a) T. It refers to the unconscious process of taking on
        some of the activities or characteristics of another
        person.
    (b) F. In sublimation, the anxieties become channelled into
        positive acts or ways of life.
    (c) F. It is a means of dealing with uncomfortable emotions
        or attributes by resisting acknowledgment of them
        within oneself and by attributing them to others.
    (d) F. It is characterized by warding off an unacceptable
        wish or impulse by adopting a character trait that is
        diametrically opposed to it.
    (e) F.
    'Conversion' of psychic energy into physical channels and
    'repression' are other mental mechanisms involved in
    hysteria-dissociative states.

40. (a) T.
    (b) T.
    (c) F. Broadmann distinguished 47 regions of cerebral
        cortex on the basis of differences in their cellular
        architecture. Many of these were subsequently
        identified as functional units, including the motor
        cortex, premotor cortex, visual cortex, auditory
        cortex, somatosensory cortex etc.
    (d) F. It is, in fact, a sheet of grey matter.
    (e) T. The Martinotti cells are modified stellate cells and
        together with stellate cells form vertical connections
        within the cerebral cortex.

41. (a) F. In thyrotoxicosis, there is weight loss despite increased appetite.
    (b) T. Up to about half of anorexics have episodes of uncontrollable over-eating, sometimes called binge eating or bulimia.
    (c) F. The Kleine–Levin syndrome consists of somnolence and increased appetite, often lasting for days or weeks and with long periods of normality between them.
    (d) F.
    (e) F.

42. (a) T.
    (b) T.
    (c) F. Anticholinergic drugs produce relaxation of bronchi.
    (d) F. They lead to reduced gastric secretion
    (e) T.

43. (a) F. Malingering is the voluntary production and presentation of false or grossly exaggerated physical or psychological symptoms. The symptoms are produced in pursuit of a goal that is obviously recognizable with an understanding of the individual's circumstances rather than of his or her individual psychology.
    (b) T.
    (c) T.
    (d) T.
    (e) F. An awareness of change is present which is lacking in dissociative disorders.

44. (a) F.
    (b) F. There may be diffuse irregularity and excess fast activity.
    (c) F.
    (d) T.
    (e) F. The EEG is often, but not invariably, of reduced amplitude.

45. (a) F.
    (b) T.
    (c) T.
    (d) T.
    (e) T.
    The 'core psychopathology' of anorexia nervosa and
    bulimia nervosa comprises a characteristic set of
    overvalued ideas concerning shape and weight which
    appear to be of major importance in maintaining these
    eating disorders. The body image disturbance is one of the
    least well understood aspects of these disorders. It includes
    body shape misperception (all or some parts of body are
    seen as larger than their actual size) and body shape
    disparagement (an intense dislike of the body or parts of
    it). One of the features which distinguishes bulimia nervosa
    from anorexia nervosa is the profound loss of control over
    eating.

46. (a) F.
    (b) F. Moclobemide should be avoided in severe hepatic
        impairment.
    (c) F.
    (d) T.
    (e) F.

47. (a) T.
    (b) T.
    (c) T.
    (d) T. Most depressed patients complain of loss of appetite.
        However, some patients eat more and gain weight. It
        seems that eating brings temporary relief to their
        distressing feelings.
    (e) F.

48. (a) T.
    (b) F.
    (c) T.
    (d) F.
    (e) T.
    Misidentification may occur in confusional states and
    schizophrenia. It may be both positive and negative.
    In Capgras' syndrome the patient believes that a person
    closely related to him or her has been replaced by a double.
    In negative misidentification the patient denies that his or
    her friends and relatives are the people whom they say they
    are and insists that they are strangers in disguise. In
    schizophrenia, it can be based on a delusional perception.
    It could also result from an excessive concretization of
    memory images, so that the person retains all the minute
    details of the characteristics of the people whom he or she
    encounters. When he or she sees the same person again,
    he/she compares the new perception with the exact
    memory image.

49. (a) T. A neurone or nerve cell consists of a cell body or
             soma, known as perikaryon or neurocyte, and
             neurites – axons and dendrites.
    (b) T. The other structures include the nucleolus, Nissl
             substance, Golgi apparatus, mitochondria,
             microfilaments, microtubules and lysosomes.
    (c) F. Neuroglia, also known as interstitial cells, make up
             most of the nervous tissue, outnumbering neurones
             five to ten times.
    (d) F. The axon of a neurone may be ensheathed in a
             lamellated interrupted covering called the myelin
             sheath.
    (e) F. It is a gap at the junction of two neurones.

50. (a) F. It is the latent or hidden content of the dream which can be interpreted to understand the unconscious issues in the dream.
    (b) F. Secondary process thinking is conscious and is based on the reality principle.
    (c) F.
    (d) T.
    (e) F. It is the pubertal phase of psychosexual development which may lead to resurgence of sexual drives by hormonal changes.

ANSWERS TO PAPER 4

1. (a) T.
   (b) T.
   (c) T.
   (d) T.
   (e) F.
   Learning is a relatively permanent change in behaviour brought about as a result of prior experience. Learning may occur through associations being made between two or more phenomena. Three types of learning theories: associative learning (classical and operant conditioning), cognitive learning and social learning theory, are recognized.

2. (a) T.
   (b) F.
   (c) T.
   (d) F.
   (e) F.
   Falsification of memory with persecutory content occurs in schizophrenia but is not considered to be a frequent feature.

3. (a) F. It is considered to be due to inhibition of presynaptic reuptake of 5-hydroxytryptamine.
   (b) F. Drug–receptor interactions may be modified by changes in receptor sensitivity. After prolonged stimulation of cells by agonists the cell becomes refractory to further stimulation. This is termed as 'down regulation' or 'desensitization'.
   (c) T.
   (d) F.
   (e) T.

4. (a) F.
   (b) F. It is a feature of a cerebellar disorder.
   (c) F.
   (d) T.
   (e) T.
   The characteristic features of generalized anxiety disorder
   are broadly grouped into four categories: motor tension,
   autonomic hyperactivity, apprehensive expectation and
   problems with vigilance and scanning.

5. (a) F. The correct term is arbitrary inference, which
          includes making conclusions based on inadequate
          information.
   (b) F. The term is overgeneralization, wherein the person is
          is likely to make sweeping judgements based on
          single instances.
   (c) F. The term is actually selective abstraction, where
          attention is paid only to negative aspects of an
          experience.
   (d) T. In dichotomous reasoning the person tends to think
          in terms of extremes.
   (e) F.

6. (a) F.
   (b) T.
   (c) T.
   (d) T.
   (e) T.
   Denial is a form of defence against anxiety and it refers to
   the inability of the individual to acknowledge some reality.

7. (a) T.
   (b) F. The afferent fibres bypass the lateral geniculate
          bodies and pass medially to the superior colliculi.
   (c) T.
   (d) F. The afferent fibres never reach the occipital cortex
          but end in the oculomotor nuclei from where the
          efferent path originates.
   (e) T.

8. (a) F.
   (b) T.
   (c) F.
   (d) T. Anorexics are usually alert, even though they are emaciated.
   (e) T. Except in longstanding cases, appetite for food persists and, for this reason, the term anorexia is a misnomer.

9. (a) F.
   (b) T.
   (c) T.
   (d) F.
   (e) T.
   Open-ended questions encourage the patient to mention his or her main problems. The interviewer should begin history-taking by asking an open-ended question.

10. (a) T.
    (b) T.
    (c) T.
    (d) F.
    (e) T.
    To make a diagnosis of depression there should be presence of depressed mood, anhedonia or increased fatigability or all three. Other symptoms are also important in making such a diagnosis, e.g. reduced self-esteem and self-confidence, ideas of guilt and unworthiness, ideas or acts of self-harm, diminished appetite etc.

11. (a) F. The word 'neurosis' is discarded by both DSMIIIR and DSMIV. The disorders previously thought to be 'neuroses' are described as anxiety disorders, somatoform disorders, factitious disorders and dissociative disorders etc.
    (b) F. As in (a).
    (c) T. Hypochondriasis is included in somatoform disorders.
    (d) F. It is a type of personality disorder on Axis II.
    (e) F. There is no separate category of late paraphrenia under schizophrenia and other psychotic disorders.

12. (a) F.
    (b) F.
    (c) F.
    (d) T.
    (e) F. Highly polar water-soluble, non-lipid-soluble drugs and proteins have a low rate of penetration through the blood–brain barrier.

13. (a) T.
    (b) T.
    (c) T. Pheochromocytomas are a rare and easily overlooked cause of episodic attacks of anxiety. However, depression may be a presenting symptom.
    (d) T. The presentation of Alzheimer's disease is often with minor forgetfulness, which is difficult to distinguish from normal ageing. The mood may be predominantly depressed, euphoric, flattened or labile.
    (e) T.

14. (a) T. Chlorpromazine inhibits hepatic enzymes which may result in reduced metabolism of the tricyclic antidepressant drugs, leading to their higher plasma levels and enhanced effects.
    (b) F.
    (c) T.
    (d) T.
    (e) T. Anticholinergic drugs slow gastric emptying, leading to delay in their systemic absorption.

15. (a) F.
    (b) T.
    (c) T.
    (d) T.
    (e) T.
    The mental symptoms may accompany pernicious anaemia and subacute combined degeneration of the spinal cord or precede them by many months.

16. (a) F. The conscious aspect of the ego is the executive organ of the psyche, responsible for decision making and integration of perceptual data. The unconscious aspect of ego contains defence mechanisms which are necessary to counteract the powerful instinctual drives harboured in the id.
    (b) T. It is only interested in discharging tension. It is controlled by both the unconscious aspects of the ego and the superego.
    (c) T. Secondary process thinking is logical, rational and geared to meet the demands of the real world.
    (d) T. It represents all the inherited, biological and constitutional features of the basic drives such as aggression, eating, sex and elimination.
    (e) F. The superego is built up from internalized representations of the standards and ideals upheld by others who are particularly important to us.

17. (a) T.
    (b) T.
    (c) F. Standardized rating scales are useful but not necessary in day-to-day clinical practice.
    (d) F. During an interview the patient may give hints of important problems or feelings by changes in tone, facial expression or posture. The interviewer should be alert to this possibility and pursue such cues by commenting on them.
    (e) T. As in (d).

18. (a) T.
    (b) T.
    (c) T.
    (d) F. It may also occur in dominant temporal lobe lesions.
    (e) F. As in (d).
    The other features include hemisomatognosia, prosopagnosia, psychotic symptomatology, epilepsy. However, the last two symptoms are not specific to non-dominant temporal lobe.

19. (a) T.
    (b) F.
    (c) F.
    (d) T.
    (e) F.
    The term late paraphrenia is sometimes used as an omnibus
    term to describe paranoid illnesses presenting for the first
    time in middle or old age. A high proportion of these
    patients are unmarried, divorced or widowed, with a
    female preponderance. These people are sensitive, jealous,
    opinionated, puritanical or self-centred. Deafness is
    common.

20. (a) T.
    (b) F. L-Dopa is a dopamine agonist drug used for the
        treatment of primary Parkinsonism.
    (c) T.
    (d) T.
    (e) T.

21. (a) F. Drowsiness but not sedation is one of the common
        side-effects of phenelzine.
    (b) T. Sedation is one of the commonest side-effects due to
        noradrenergic and histaminergic action of the
        antidepressant drug.
    (c) T. As in (b).
    (d) F. Drowsiness but not sedation is a common side-effect.
    (e) F. As in (d).

22. (a) T. It is proposed that anxiety is experienced for the first time during the process of birth (primary anxiety).
    (b) F. It is linked with depression.
    (c) T. During the Oedipal phase, anxiety focuses on potential damage to or loss of the genitals of a retaliatory parental figure.
    (d) T. It is thought that the child is overwhelmed by stimulation at the very moment of separation from its mother. It has been suggested that this may explain why separation can provoke anxiety.
    (e) F. It is linked with depression.

Anxiety is an affect that was instrumental to the birth of psychoanalysis and psychodynamic psychiatry. Freud considered anxiety as both a symptomatic manifestation of neurotic conflict as well as an adaptive signal to ward off awareness of neurotic conflict.

23. (a) F. Mitochondria are present throughout the neurone and are involved in energy production. Dendrites also contain Nissl substance which synthesizes protein.
    (b) F. Dendrites like the cell body and axon hillock of the neurone are unmyelinated.
    (c) F. They are found in both central nervous system (brain and spinal cord) and peripheral nervous system (cranial and spinal nerves and other neuronal processes).
    (d) T. The dendritic spines form the subsynaptic membrane (synaptic plates) of the axodendritic synapses.
    (e) T.

24. (a) F. According to Schneider, the presence of one or more first rank symptoms in the absence of organic disease can be used as positive evidence for schizophrenia.
    (b) T.
    (c) F.
    (d) F.
    (e) T. It means audible thoughts (*echo de la pensées* in French), i.e. the patient hears his or her own thoughts said out loud.

25. (a) T.
    (b) F. In multiaxial classification, the clinical syndrome is
        recorded on Axis I. Other axes allow the systematic
        recording of different information sets.
    (c) T.
    (d) T.
    (e) F. Diagnostic reliability is considerably higher using
        structured and standardized interviews than is
        possible with unstructured interviews.

26. (a) T.
    (b) T.
    (c) T.
    (d) T.
    (e) F.
    Frank Fish and Hughlings Jackson in the 19th century used
    to distinguish between positive and negative symptoms, on
    the basis of reduction or loss of normal cerebral function.
    Poverty of speech and loosening of association are the
    other negative symptoms of schizophrenia.

27. (a) F. Axillary and pubic hair are preserved and there is no
        breast atrophy.
    (b) F. Body weight is maintained at least 15% below that
        expected, or Quetelet's body-mass index is 17.5 or
        less.
    (c) T. In about a fifth of cases, amenorrhoea precedes
        weight loss.
    (d) T. A fine downy lanugo hair is sometimes found on the
        back, arms and sides of the face.
    (e) T. It is a male equivalent to amenorrhoea.
    Quetelet's body-mass index = weight $(kg)/(height (m))^2$

28. (a) T.
    (b) T.
    (c) T.
    (d) T.
    (e) T.
    The above include some of the common and likely causes
    of sexual dysfunction.

29. (a) F.
   (b) F. Cataplexy – sudden loss of muscle tone – is one of the main features of polysymptomatic narcolepsy.
   (c) F. The EEG is normal with abnormally rapid onset of REM-stage sleep during an afternoon nap or the abnormally rapid onset of stage 1 sleep during a multiple daytime EEG sleep latency test.
   (d) T. See (b).
   (e) F. In night terror, the child wakes up with intense anxiety or terror which is accompanied by complete amnesia for the experience on waking.

30. (a) F. In borderline syndrome, i.e. borderline personality disorder, there is a pervasive pattern of instability of interpersonal relationships, self-image and affects, and marked impulsivity that begins by early adulthood.
   (b) F. As in (e).
   (c) T. Pseudohallucinations are abnormal phenomena that do not meet the criteria for hallucinations (i.e. percepts experienced in the absence of an external stimulus to the sense organs, and with a similar quality to a true percept). Pseudohallucinations are figurative and always located in subjective space and perceived with the inner eye or ear.
   (d) F. True hallucinations may occur in healthy people, especially when tired.
   (e) F. Hypnagogic and hypnopompic hallucinations may be visual, auditory or tactile. They occur while falling asleep and during awakening respectively.

31. (a) T. Wernicke's encephalopathy is caused by severe deficiency of thiamine (vitamin B1). The other features include ophthalmoplegia, and clouding of consciousness.
   (b) T. As in (a).
   (c) F.
   (d) T.
   (e) F. It is associated with vitamin B12 deficiency.

32 (a) F. Imprinting – an ethological concept – leads to
attachment behaviour learned during a critical
period of life.
   (b) F. Learned helplessness, which consists of a belief that
one has no control over the environment and
reduced voluntary movement, occurs in depression.
   (c) T.
   (d) T.
   (e) F.

33. (a) F.
    (b) T.
    (c) T.
    (d) F.
    (e) F.
Before the interview begins, the interviewer should ensure
that the patient knows the exact purpose of the interview
and that the setting is right.

34. (a) F. The hypothalamus contains a large variety of nuclei
which secrete a number of releasing factors for the
target cells in the pituitary gland.
    (b) T.
    (c) F. It forms the floor of the third ventricle and is made
of a number of nuclei.
    (d) T.
    (e) T.

35. (a) F.
    (b) F.
    (c) F.
    (d) F.
    (e) F.
All the above were described by Kurt Schneider.
Carl Schneider described five features of formal thought
disorder, i.e. derailment, substitution, omission, fusion
and drivelling.

36. (a) T.
    (b) T.
    (c) T.
    (d) T.
    (e) F. G proteins interact with multiple effectors.

37. (a) T. Archetypes are generalized symbols and images
        within the collective unconscious which refers to the
        myths common to all mankind.
    (b) F. It is associated with Sigmund Freud.
    (c) T. Animus is the unconscious, masculine side of the
        woman's female persona.
    (d) F. According to Adler, 'inferiority complex' is
        concerned with specific body organs either in reality
        or in fantasy.
    (e) F. The concept of 'transitional object' is associated with
        Winnicott. It is an intermediate between oral
        eroticism and true object relationships.

38. (a) F. This is an example of second person auditory
        hallucination which does not point to a particular
        diagnosis. However, its content and especially the
        patient's reaction may do so.
    (b) T. This is an example of thought broadcasting.
    (c) T. This is an example of delusional perception.
    (d) T. This is an example of a passivity of volition.
    (e) T. This is an example of thought insertion.

39. (a) F. Alpha spindles are present in stage 1, while sleep
        spindles of fast activity are present in stage 2 of
        sleep.
    (b) T. Grand mal seizures are activated in non-REM sleep,
        while absences or minor seizures may be seen in
        REM sleep.
    (c) F. This is the case with patients suffering from
        narcolepsy.
    (d) T.
    (e) T.

40. (a) T.
    (b) F. It is an azaspirodecanedione type anxiolytic drug.
    (c) F. It is a cyclopyrolone hypnotic drug.
    (d) F. It is a selective NA (Nor adrenaline) reuptake
        inhibitor antidepressant drug.
    (e) F. It is a reversible monoamine oxidase inhibitor type A
        antidepressant drug.

41. (a) T.
    (b) F. Asking direct questions about suicidal ideation or
        intent may in fact reduce the risk as the patients may
        feel relieved.
    (c) F.
    (d) F. Denial of suicide intent does not necessarily imply a
        high risk. The most obvious warning sign is a direct
        statement of intent. About two-thirds of those who
        die by suicide have told someone of their intention.
    (e) T.

42. (a) F.
    (b) F.
    (c) F.
    (d) F.
    (e) F.
    The dopamine-containing fibres originate in nucleus A10
    and innervate olfactory tubercle, septal nuclei (lateral
    septal nucleus and nucleus accumbens), interstitial cells of
    the stria terminalis, cingulate cortex and oral part of
    parahippocampal cortex.

43. (a) T.
    (b) T.
    (c) T.
    (d) F.
    (e) F.
    Obsessions are recurrent, persistent thoughts, impulses or
    images that enter the mind despite the person's efforts to
    exclude them. They are often regarded by the person as his
    or her own, untrue or senseless. They are generally about
    matters which the patient finds distressing or unpleasant.

44. (a) F.
    (b) F. Drowsiness but not sedation is one of the
         commonest side-effects.
    (c) F. As in (b).
    (d) F. Drowsiness but not sedation is a common side-effect
         in therapeutic dosage of nortriptyline.
    (e) F.

45. (a) F. The concept of free association is associated with
         Sigmund Freud.
    (b) T. 'Persona' is the front we present to the world.
    (c) T. 'Anima' is the unconscious feminine side of the
         man's male persona.
    (d) F. It is linked with Melanie Klein. It is the realization
         that mother is both good and bad which leads to guilt
         and fear of destroying the loved one with the hatred.
    (e) F.

46. (a) T.
    (b) F.
    (c) T.
    (d) F.
    (e) F.

47. (a) T.
    (b) F. It involves alternating translations of electrical
         signals into chemical messages, through
         neurotransmitters, and of chemical messages into
         electrical signals.
    (c) T.
    (d) F. The synapse acts as a one-way valve allowing
         transmission of nerve impulses in one direction only.
    (e) T.

48. (a) T.
    (b) T.
    (c) T.
    (d) T.
    (e) F. The patient may exhibit a blunted or flattened affect.
    When emotions change in an excessively rapid and abrupt
    way, the affect is said to be labile.

49. (a) F.
    (b) T.
    (c) T.
    (d) T.
    (e) T.
    According to psychoanalytic theory, anxiety is viewed as
    the result of 'psychic conflict' between unconscious sexual
    or aggressive wishes stemming from the id and
    corresponding threats of punishment from the superego.

50. (a) F. The main feature of somatoform disorders is
        repeated presentation of physical symptoms,
        together with persistent requests for medical
        investigations, in spite of repeated negative findings
        and reassurances by doctors that the symptoms have
        no physical basis.
    (b) T. It is a rare disorder characterized by the
        'approximate answers', usually accompanied by
        several other dissociative symptoms.
    (c) F. Neurasthenia is characterized by either persistent
        and distressing complaints of increased fatigue after
        mental effort or the same complaints of bodily
        weakness and exhaustion after minimal physical
        effort.
    (d) T. It is a rare disorder characterized by the apparent
        existence of two or more distinct personalities within
        an individual, with only one of them being evident at
        a given time.
    (e) F. The essential features of hypochondriasis include a
        persistent preoccupation with the possibility of
        having one or more serious and progressive physical
        disorders.

ANSWERS TO PAPER 5

1. (a) F.
   (b) T.
   (c) T.
   (d) F.
   (e) T.
   The signs of lithium intoxication are blurred vision,
   increasing gastrointestinal disturbances (anorexia,
   vomiting, diarrhoea), coarse tremor, lack of co-ordination,
   dysarthria, nystagmus and convulsions. The treatment
   should be stopped immediately, plasma-lithium
   concentrations redetermined and steps should be taken to
   reverse lithium toxicity.

2. (a) F. Only positron emission tomography can be used for
   in-vivo receptor imaging.
   (b) T.
   (c) F. Clozapine occupancy is only partial (37%) whereas
   it is 85% with haloperidol.
   (d) T.
   (e) F. Labelled flumazenil is used for benzodiazepine
   receptors.

3. (a) F. Pareidolia is a type of illusion in which real and unreal percepts exist side by side, the latter being recognized as unreal. It occurs, without making any effort, in normal people. It can also occur in acute organic disorder.

   (b) T. It consists of senseless omission of a thought or part of it.

   (c) T. They refer to two words with a similar sound which are used to preserve the ordinary logical sequence of ideas. Clang associations occur in poetry and in humour and also in manic speech where the clang occurs on the terminal syllable.

   (d) T. It is a Schneider's first rank symptom in which the patient hears his own thoughts out loud. He knows that they are his own thoughts, yet he hears them audibly either while he is thinking them, just before, or just after.

   (e) T. It is a type of loosening of associations. It refers to a transition from one topic to another, either between sentences or in mid-sentence with no logical relationship between the two topics. It is also known as Knight's move.

4. (a) F. It was published in 1992 by The World Health Oganization (WHO).

   (b) T.

   (c) F.

   (d) F. See (a).

   (e) F. The traditional division between neurosis and psychosis has not been used but the term 'neurotic' is still retained for occasional use in categories F40–F48.

5. (a) F. Confrontation with the patient may lead to irritable and unco-operative behaviour on the part of the patient.

   (b) F. One should be neutral in approaching the paranoid delusions.

   (c) T.

   (d) T.

   (e) T.

6. (a) T. They are intracellular paired helical filaments seen in the hippocampus, amygdala, neocortex, locus coeruleus, nucleus of Meynert, and raphe nuclei.
   (b) F. They are characterized by the deposition of Beta A4 protein in the extracellular space, which is an abnormal fragment of the amyloid precursor protein, the gene for which is on chromosome 21.
   (c) T.
   (d) F. Ependyma are a type of interstitial brain cell which make up most of the nervous tissue. Other cells include astrocytes, oligodendrocytes and microglia.
   (e) T.

7. (a) F.
   (b) T.
   (c) T.
   (d) T.
   (e) T. Other schedules of reinforcement include: continuous reinforcement, mixed interval, variable interval, mixed ratio and variable ratio reinforcement.
   In behaviour therapy, emphasis is placed not on diagnosing syndromes but on discovering current factors related to the problem. The treatment is only given after a detailed examination of the precise circumstances surrounding the problem, i.e. functional behavioural analysis.

8. (a) F. Although cognitive theory does not specifically address the first attack, it is thought that most panic attacks occur as a result of a tendency to catastrophically misinterpret bodily sensations.
   (b) T. Avoidance helps by reinforcing the person's belief that something disastrous was prevented from happening by his or her actions.
   (c) F. Any stimulus that is perceived as threatening either external or internal can lead to a panic attack.
   (d) F.
   (e) F. Although to an extent this response may seem correct, the crucial factor is the person believing that something catastrophic is about to happen immediately.

9. (a) F.
 (b) T.
 (c) F.
 (d) F.
 (e) T.

10. (a) F. D2 receptor antagonists are believed to possess antipsychotic activity.
 (b) T.
 (c) F. Benzodiazepines act directly by binding with benzodiazepine receptors which are themselves linked to GABA receptors in an ionophore or complex involving GABA, benzodiazepine receptors and a chloride channel. In addition, they block cortical arousal, which occurs after stimulation of the mid-brain reticular activity system.
 (d) F. Its mode of action in treatment of affective disorders has not been identified. It is postulated that lithium stimulates sodium and magnesium dependent adenosine triphosphatase (ATP-ase), inhibits adenyl cyclase and inositol phosphate intracellular secondary messenger systems throughout the body and in brain by altering the functions of guanosine triphosphate (GTP)-binding proteins.
 (e) F. Its action appears to be mediated through $5\text{-HT}_1 A$ receptors, where it is a partial agonist, and D2 receptors to which it weakly binds.

11. (a) T.
 (b) T.
 (c) T.
 (d) T.
 (e) T. Computerized tomography is used extensively in clinical practice. It is able to demonstrate shifts of intracranial structures and expanding intracranial lesions. It has also proved to be a useful psychiatric research tool.

12. (a) T.
    (b) T.
    (c) F.
    (d) T.
    (e) T.

13. (a) T. Although life events seem to have an effect, the size
        of the effect is uncertain.
    (b) F. None of the theories of disordered communication
        within a family can give a satisfactory explanation
        why it is unusual for more than one child in a family
        to develop schizophrenia.
    (c) F. A double-bind is said to occur when an instruction is
        given overtly but contradicted by a second, more
        covert instruction.
    (d) F. The dopamine hypothesis indicates that there is a
        dopamine overactivity in the mesolimbic system.
    (e) T. Retrospective studies of schizophrenic patients
        report more obstetric complications than do studies
        of normal controls.

14. (a) F. It regulates the movement of substances into and out
        of the nervous system.
    (b) T.
    (c) F.
    (d) T. Lipid-soluble substances pass readily through the
        membrane, while non-lipid-soluble substances and
        proteins enter the brain very slowly.
    (e) T. This states that the permeability of a cell membrane
        to a drug is proportional to that drug's partition
        parameter. The latter is the product of two fractional
        concentrations, one of the un-ionized drug in
        aqueous solution and the other the lipid solubility of
        the un-ionized drug.

15. (a) T.
    (b) F.
    (c) T.
    (d) F.
    (e) T.

16. (a) F.
    (b) T.
    (c) F.
    (d) F.
    (e) F.
    A few patients accustomed to a fairly high dose of a tricyclic antidepressant drug will experience a withdrawal syndrome if the drug is abruptly withdrawn. This syndrome is characterized by malaise, headache, nausea, abdominal pain, diarrhoea and restlessness. It is caused by cholinergic hyperfunction.

17. (a) T. Obsessional ruminations are repeated worrying themes of a complex kind, e.g. about the ending of the world.
    (b) T. Rituals, i.e. compulsions, are usually associated with obsessions if they have the function of reducing the distress caused by the latter.
    (c) F. This refers to compulsive rituals.
    (d) F. A prodrome of non-specific symptoms appears in some young people. It includes symptoms such as loss of interest, avoiding the company of others, staying away from work, irritability and oversensitivity.
    (e) T.

18. (a) F. The EEG is similar to that of the relaxed wakeful state.
    (b) F. EEG maturation both in the foetus and throughout life involves frequency and wave form changes.
    (c) F. The EEG changes are similar to those observed with tricyclic antidepressants such as slowing of the alpha wave and increasing slow wave activity.
    (d) T.
    (e) T.

19. (a) F. Sublimation is a mature or healthy ego defence mechanism.
    (b) F. It is associated with latency phase of psychosexual development.
    (c) F. As in (a).
    (d) F. See item (e) in the question.
    (e) T.

20. (a) F. The essential feature of social phobia is a marked and persistent fear of social or performance situations in which embarrassment may occur.
    (b) T. The other symptoms of social phobia include palpitations, tremors, sweating, gastrointestinal discomfort, diarrhoea, muscle tension and confusion.
    (c) F. The patient typically avoids the feared situations.
    (d) F.
    (e) T. Some patients take alcohol to relieve the symptoms of anxiety. Alcohol abuse is more common in social phobias than in other phobias.

21. (a) T.
    (b) T.
    (c) T.
    (d) T.
    (e) F. Usually, patients who are dependent on alcohol take the first drink in the morning to control tremor as well as other withdrawal symptoms.

22. (a) T.
    (b) T.
    (c) F.
    (d) T.
    (e) F.

23. (a) F.
    (b) T.
    (c) T.
    (d) F.
    (e) T.
    The features of motor neurone disease include: difficulty in swallowing, chewing, coughing, breathing and talking, wasted and fasciculating tongue, muscle stiffness and weakness. There are no objective changes on sensory examination.

24. (a) T.
    (b) T.
    (c) T.
    (d) T.
    (e) F.
    Because of the limited capacity of our information-processing system, it is essential that we are able to restrict the total input to a manageable amount. It is also necessary to ensure that important information is allowed through for processing while the irrelevant and unimportant is screened out.

    In dissociative states, it is presumed that the ability to exercise a conscious and selective control is impaired. Similar mechanisms may operate in (b), (c) and (d).

25. (a) F. Both (a) and (e) are the principal components of the corpus striatum of the basal ganglia. The corpus striatum is important in control of posture and initiation of movement, and is probably involved in the balance between alpha and gamma motor neurone activity.
    (b) T.
    (c) T.
    (d) T The hypothalamus acts as a control centre for the regulation of the internal environment.
    (e) F. As in (a).

26. (a) F. Perseveration usually occurs in association with disturbance of memory. It is defined as a response that was appropriate to a first stimulus being given inappropriately to a second, different stimulus. It is a sign of organic brain disease.

(b) F. It is a disorder of the stream of thought. Here ideas arise in unusual variety and abundance and pass through the mind rapidly.

(c) F. It is a disorder of the stream of thought. Here the patient has only a few thoughts, which lack variety and richness and seem to move through the mind slowly.

(d) F. Confabulation is a falsification of memory occurring in clear consciousness in association with an organically derived amnesia.

(e) F. It is disorder of tempo of thinking in which there is no general direction of thinking and the connections between successive thought appear to be due to chance factors which can usually be understood.

27. (a) T. Near-death experience is a complex hallucinatory phenomenon in people who perceive death as imminent. It seems to be comparable to other mental reactions to perceived threat, coloured by culture and current stress.

(b) T. Pseudohallucinations are a type of mental image which, although clear and vivid, lack the substantiality of perceptions. They are seen in full consciousness, known not to be real perceptions and are not located in objective space but in subjective space.

(c) T. Ideas of reference are held by people who are unduly self-conscious. The person realizes that this feeling originates within him/herself. They may be present in many psychiatric disorders.

(d) T.

(e) T. In delusional mood, the patient has the knowledge that there is something going on around him/her which concerns him/her but he/she does not know what it is. Usually the meaning of delusional mood becomes apparent when a sudden delusional perception occurs.

28. (a) T.
    (b) T.
    (c) T.
    (d) T.
    (e) F.
    Neurotoxic effects may be acute or chronic. Potential
    mechanisms of neurotoxicity are legion. They include
    selective interference with basic metabolic processes, protein
    and nucleic acid synthesis, nerve membrane permeability or
    synaptic transmission. The clinical picture includes
    symptoms of severe motor, mental and autonomic disorders.

29. (a) F. 'Epinosic' means secondary to all illness, i.e. it refers
        to a secondary gain.
    (b) F. The patient may exercise considerable control over
        his or her environment, including people around him
        or her.
    (c) T.
    (d) T.
    (e) T.

30. (a) T.
    (b) F. Such an activity is a normal feature of sleep.
    (c) F. Opening the eyes leads to alpha blocking,
        i.e. replacement of alpha activity by beta activity.
    (d) T.
    (e) F. In fact they vary with age in human beings.

31. (a) T.
    (b) T.
    (c) T.
    (d) T.
    (e) T.
    Abnormal perceptions are divided into:
    (i) sensory distortions where a real perceptual object is
        perceived distorted; and
    (ii) false perceptions, where a new perception occurs which
        may or may not be in response to an external stimulus.
        They include illusions, hallucinations and
        pseudohallucinations.

32. (a) F. Receptor recognition sites occur at synapses.
    (b) F. Life span of receptors varies from 7 to 30 days.
    (c) F. Receptors are synthesized in the cell body and then transported down the axon into the target sites on the cell membrane.
    (d) T.
    (e) T.

33. (a) F. It is a disorder of muscle tone in which the patient allows him/herself to be placed in an awkward posture which he/she then maintains apparently without distress for much longer than most people could achieve without severe discomfort.
    (b) T. Somnambulism, i.e. sleep walking, usually occurs in children, and in males more often than females. Activity is usually confined to aimless wandering and purposeless repetitive behaviour for a few minutes.
    (c) F. Night terrors occur in deep sleep early in the night and often in the individual who also sleep walks. Intense anxiety is manifested. Usually there is complete amnesia for the experience on waking.
    (d) F. In cataplexy, the subject falls down due to sudden loss of muscle tone provoked by strong emotion.
    (e) T.
    The common theme shared by dissociative states is a partial or complete loss of the normal integration between memories of the past, awareness of identity and immediate sensations and control of bodily movements. All types of dissociative states tend to remit after a few weeks or months.

34. (a) T.
    (b) F. The patient's relationship to the therapist is a
        mixture of a transference relationship and a real
        relationship. This latter relationship is termed the
        therapeutic alliance or the working alliance. As part
        of the working alliance, the patient must achieve a
        realistic view of the treatment programme.
    (c) T.
    (d) T.
    (e) F. As in (b).

35. (a) T.
    (b) T.
    (c) F. It is a lamellated interrupted membrane covering the
        axon of a nerve cell.
    (d) T.
    (e) T.
    The blood–brain barrier is responsible for preventing rapid
    equilibration of some drugs between the blood, on one
    hand, and the brain and cerebrospinal fluid, on the other
    hand. The normal operation of the blood–brain barrier
    may alter in presence of acute cerebral lesions, e.g.
    infection.

36. (a) T. It supplies the inferior half of the anterior limb.
    (b) T. It supplies the superior halves of the anterior and
        posterior limbs.
    (c) F.
    (d) T. It supplies the posterior two-thirds of the posterior
        limb.
    (e) T. The posterior communicating branch of the internal
        carotid artery supplies the anterior one-third of the
        posterior limb of the internal capsule.

37. (a) T.
    (b) T.
    (c) T.
    (d) T.
    (e) T.
    Antimuscarinic drugs exert their anti-Parkinsonian effect
    by correcting the relative central cholinergic excess thought
    to occur in Parkinsonism as a result of dopamine
    deficiency. Their unwanted effects include gastrointestinal
    disturbances, dizziness, blurred vision, urinary retention,
    tachycardia, nervousness and excitement.

38. (a) F.
    (b) T.
    (c) T.
    (d) T.
    (e) T.
    From a psychodynamic perspective, the term 'schizoid'
    reflects a splitting or fragmentation of the self into different
    self-representations that remain unintegrated. The result is
    a diffuse identity, i.e. the schizoid patients are not sure   —
    who they are.

39. (a) T.
    (b) T.
    (c) F. The patient has limited capacity to express either
             warm, tender feelings or anger towards others.
    (d) F. The patient is apparently indifferent to either praise
             or criticism.
    (e) F. The patient exhibits excessive preoccupation with
             fantasy and introspection. He or she also shows
             marked insensitivity to prevailing social norms and
             conventions.

40. (a) F.
    (b) T. Where the aetiology is uncertain, it is justifiable to combine physically oriented measures and psychological techniques such as behaviour therapy or psychotherapy.
    (c) F.
    (d) T.
    (e) F.

Spasmodic torticollis is a rare condition in which there are repeated, purposeless movements of the head and neck or sustained abnormal positions or both. Its causes include organic or psychogenic factors or both. Its treatment is unsatisfactory.

41. (a) T.
    (b) T.
    (c) F. It includes the subject's overt responses such as avoidance, escape behaviours and ritualistic behaviours. Operational definitions of these responses are not usually included.
    (d) T.
    (e) F. It consists of a highly detailed account of current determinants of the problem. Behaviour therapy is interested in the perpetuating factors.

42. (a) T.
    (b) T.
    (c) T.
    (d) T.
    (e) F.

There are several processes that maintain bulimia nervosa once it is established. Overconcern drives dieting; the dieting in turn is likely to encourage binges, which are also encouraged by the purgative and diuretic abuse, as well as by self-induced vomiting. The binges undermine the patient's sense of self-control and self-esteem, thus exacerbating feelings of ineffectiveness and intensifying concern with shape and weight.

43. (a) T.
    (b) T.
    (c) F.
    (d) T.
    (e) F.
    The placebo-effect refers to the fact that any treatment will produce beneficial results if given or taken with enough faith and enthusiasm. It is dependent on a number of factors such as the nature and quantity of the placebo preparation given, the situation and manner in which it is given, the social and psychological attributes of the recipient, the condition being treated etc.

44. (a) T. Most diagnoses have an empirical literature or available data sets that are relevant to decisions regarding the revision of the diagnostic manual.
    (b) T.
    (c) T.
    (d) T. It retains two kinds of hierarchy: organic mental disorder pre-empts the diagnosis of any disorder that could produce part of the symptomatology, and schizophrenia pre-empts other disorders in the same way.
    (e) T. It involves an assessment on several axes, each of which refers to a different domain of information that may help the clinician plan treatment and predict outcome.

45. (a) F.
    (b) F.
    (c) T. It provides the afferent path of the corneal reflex.
    (d) T. It provides the efferent path of the corneal reflex.
    (e) T. Along with the spinal nucleus of facial nerve, it provides the central path in neurotransmission.

46. (a) T.
    (b) F. One of the most serious drawbacks is that these disorders may be overlooked or misrepresented.
    (c) F. In fact, the dimensional classification system is more flexible than the categorical classification.
    (d) F. It is based on subject matter which is divided into a number of separate and mutually exclusive categories.
    (e) T.

47. (a) T.
    (b) F. It consists of ascending noradrenergic, dopaminergic and serotonergic fibres terminating in higher brain areas.
    (c) T.
    (d) T.
    (e) T.

48. (a) T. The ego corresponds to the conscious level of functioning. It develops progressively from birth. Its first task is to distinguish between the inner world of subjective experience and external reality.
    (b) T.
    (c) F. It is a concept used by Freudian analysts.
    (d) T.
    (e) T. As it is reality oriented it has to find acceptable and appropriate ways of satisfying the demands of the id, which may involve their delayed gratification.

49. (a) T. When the patient is very disturbed or suffering from organic brain disease, the mental state examination is more crucial, as it is not possible to take a history from the patient.
    (b) T. The initial questions should be as wide and as open-ended as possible.
    (c) F.
    (d) T.
    (e) T.

50. (a) F. Capgras' syndrome was first described by Capgras
        and Reboul-Lachaux in 1923. It is strictly speaking a
        single symptom and not a syndrome, namely, the
        belief that a person closely related to the patient has
        been replaced by an identical double. He or she
        accepts that the misidentified person has a great
        resemblance to the familiar person, but still believes
        that they are different people.

   (b) F. As in (a).

   (c) F. Free association is one of the psychoanalytic
        techniques.

   (d) T.

   (e) T. It is also associated with affective disorders as well as
        organic disorders.

ANSWERS TO PAPER 6

1. (a) T. In some cases the obsessions may be so bizarre that they may be difficult to distinguish from psychotic states.
   (b) T. By definition obsessions cannot be ego-alien.
   (c) F. Resistance is not invariable and is not necessary to diagnose obsessions.
   (d) F. Activities that are pleasurable are sought and are not intrusive.
   (e) T. In magical thinking, thoughts, words or actions assume power and the person believes that they can prevent events, e.g. a person may count numbers to ward off danger.

2. (a) F.
   (b) T.
   (c) F.
   (d) F. The auditory cortex receives information from both ears because the auditory pathway is not entirely crossed.
   (e) T.

3. (a) T. This is a sorting test that is sensitive to frontal lobe damage.
   (b) F. This measures intelligence and contains six verbal and five performance subtests and does not test any lobes specifically.
   (c) F. Grasp reflex tests frontal lobe dysfunction.
   (d) F. This test requires the reproduction of a series of geometrical figures and is used to detect brain damage.
   (e) F. Apraxias indicate parietal lobe damage.

4. (a) T.
   (b) F.
   (c) F.
   (d) T.
   (e) F.

5. (a) F.
   (b) F.
   (c) T.
   (d) F.
   (e) T.

Projective identification is also a projective mechanism although it is not synonymous with projection. Split-off parts of an internal object are projected into another person. Mainly bad inner objects and bad parts of the self are projected. The object is then thought of as being persecutory. It also allows making oneself understood by exerting pressure on another individual to experience feelings similar to one's own.

6. (a) F. When ill-defined subjective judgements are needed to determine presence of symptoms such as ambivalence and autism then the reliability is low.
   (b) F. Operational criteria only improve the reliability.
   (c) F. In psychiatric disorders diagnosis is based on multiple symptoms (polythetic) rather than one pathognomonic symptom (monothetic), thus lowering reliability.
   (d) F. The reasons are similar to item (a).
   (e) T. The diagnosis, at least according to the criteria in the modern classificatory systems, is based on well-defined behaviours, thus improving reliability.

7. (a) T. However, the predominant presentation is with auditory hallucinations.
   (b) F.
   (c) T.
   (d) F. One of the features that distinguishes alcoholic hallucinosis is the occurrence of hallucinations in the setting of clear consciousness. However, visual hallucinations are not prominent in alcoholic hallucinosis.
   (e) F. Can also occur with continued drinking at reduced levels.

8. (a) T.
   (b) T.
   (c) F. Four major ions; the fourth one is Ca^{++}.
   (d) F.
   (e) F. Depolarization occurs with decreased negativity.

9. (a) T.
   (b) F.
   (c) T.
   (d) T.
   (e) T.
   In somatization disorder, the aetiological factors involve contributions from several modalities, e.g. perception, cognition, affect and learnt behaviour. No relation with childhood sexual abuse has been suggested.

10. (a) T.
    (b) F.
    (c) T.
    (d) F.
    (e) T.
    Selective attention refers to the mechanisms by which only a few of the stimuli which we perceive are further processed. Broadbent described three types of processing involved. In filtering, stimuli are selected on the basis of a single distinctive physical feature. In categorizing, attention is paid to features of a stimulus which show that it belongs to a certain stimulus class. In pigeonholing, a bias is applied while attending and stimulus is selected with less perceptual evidence than would normally be needed.

11. (a) F. Seligman is associated with the concept of learned helplessness.
    (b) T.
    (c) T.
    (d) T. Donald Klein introduced the treatment of panic disorder with imipramine.
    (e) F.

12. (a) T.
    (b) T.
    (c) T.
    (d) T.
    (e) T.

13. (a) F. It consists of three layers.
    (b) T.
    (c) T. Pyramidal cells, stellate cells, multiform cells, cells of Martinotti and the horizontal cells of Cajal.
    (d) F. It is part of the archicortex.
    (e) F. They form the most superficial layer.

14. (a) T.
    (b) T.
    (c) F.
    (d) T.
    (e) T.
    A diagnosis of depression is made as long as the patient currently satisfies the criteria for depression. Obsessions can occur in depression and depression occurs commonly in those who suffer from obsessions. First rank symptoms have been described with depression. In the DSMIIIR, if the patient meets the criteria for obsessive compulsive disorder then it can be diagnosed as well on Axis I. First rank symptoms can be described as mood incongruent delusions and hallucinations.

15. (a) T. It consists of numerous microcystic spaces scattered throughout the grey matter, giving the brain a spongy appearance.
    (b) T.
    (c) F. This pathological feature is found in Wernicke–Korsakoff syndrome.
    (d) T.
    (e) F. They are present in the basal ganglia and substantia nigra of patients with Parkinson's disease and have also been found in a condition known as senile dementia of Lewy body type.

16. (a) T. Primary association areas are adjacent to the sensory areas and give rise to projections which are more widespread, and these areas are called secondary association areas.
    (b) T.
    (c) F. The primary sensory cortex receives input from the relay nuclei of the thalamus.
    (d) T.
    (e) T.

17. (a) F.
    (b) F. Subtype classified in ICD10.
    (c) T.
    (d) F.
    (e) F. A duration of six months is specified in the DSMIIIR, while in the ICD10 no specific duration is required.

18. (a) T.
    (b) T.
    (c) T.
    (d) T.
    (e) T.
    Grief may be prolonged when the situations described above occur. For example item (b): if the person has died from AIDS, then it might be difficult to acknowledge publicly.

19. (a) T.
    (b) T.
    (c) F.
    (d) T.
    (e) F.

20. (a) T.
    (b) F.
    (c) T.
    (d) F.
    (e) T.
    Ego strength refers to the capacity of an individual to effectively engage in analysis and also includes an individual's ability to regress temporarily, to be able to observe intra-psychic processes and to function responsibly in a relationship.

21. (a) F. Irritability is also a common presentation.
    (b) F.
    (c) F. Distractibility underlies the decreased attention span
        rather than any alteration of consciousness.
    (d) T. The occurrence of this symptom in the early period
        of an episode makes this a useful early warning sign.
    (e) T.

22. (a) F. Alexithymia is not a diagnosis. It has been found in
        individuals who have somatoform illnesses such as
        somatoform pain disorder.
    (b) F.
    (c) F. Alexithymia refers to an inability or difficulty of
        expressing or being aware of one's feelings or moods.
    (d) F.
    (e) F. Apart from what has been defined in answer (c),
        there are a number of features seen in people who
        have alexithymia and these include not being
        psychologically introspective or imaginative.

23. (a) F. Tachycardia has not been described as a symptom or
        a sign in depression.
    (b) T.
    (c) F.
    (d) F.
    (e) T.

24. (a) F.
    (b) F.
    (c) F.
    (d) F.
    (e) F.
    No single feature distinguishes mania from schizophrenia;
    the diagnosis is based on several symptoms occurring
    together.

25. (a) F. The description in item (a) is that of escape training.
    (b) F. This is called 'reward training'.
    (c) F. This is a description of 'avoidance training'.
    (d) F. Punitive training has not been described, although a similar experiment is conducted for learned helplessness.
    (e) F. Habitual training does not exist.

26. (a) F. Tremors occur during activity.
    (b) T.
    (c) T. However, they can occur normally during fatigue or anxiety.
    (d) F.
    (e) F. It is a combination of blepharospasm and oromandibular dyskinesia.

27. (a) T.
    (b) T.
    (c) F. It is an anticonvulsant also used in the treatment of bipolar affective disorder.
    (d) T.
    (e) T.

28. (a) F.
    (b) T.
    (c) T.
    (d) T.
    (e) F.

29. (a) F. The CAMCOG is part of the CAMDEX (Cambridge Mental Disorders of the Elderly Examination).
    (b) F. It discriminates well between delirium and dementia.
    (c) F.
    (d) F. MMPI is the Minnesota Multiphasic Personality Inventory which is a personality test.
    (e) T.

30. (a) T.
    (b) F.
    (c) T.
    (d) T.
    (e) T.
    Some of the main functions of the ego derive from its being an agency that mediates between the instinctual drives and the outside world. The capacity to form relationships that are mutually satisfying is also a very important function of the ego.

31. (a) T.
    (b) F. They can be activated both electrically and chemically. The electrically activated channels are also called 'voltage sensitive'.
    (c) T.
    (d) F.
    (e) F. Only those ion channels responsible for the action potential open when the depolarization reaches the spike threshold.

32. (a) F.
    (b) T.
    (c) T.
    (d) F.
    (e) F.

33. (a) F.
    (b) F.
    (c) F.
    (d) T.
    (e) T.

34. (a) T.
    (b) F. The relationship between depression and
        interpersonal loss is not specific as such events
        precede other disorders as well.
    (c) F. The symptom pattern of the depression does not
        appear to be strongly related to life events.
    (d) F. Such a relationship has not been found.
    (e) F. The risk of developing depression tends to fall off
        with time after the event.

35. (a) T.
    (b) T.
    (c) T.
    (d) F.
    (e) T.
    Neuropathological abnormalities are found in three-
    quarters of patients with AIDS. Besides the above
    abnormalities, focal demyelination is seen. Microscopic
    abnormalities are seen in the form of collection of
    microglia, while characteristic multinucleated cells are
    found in the white matter and subcortical grey matter.

36. (a) T.
    (b) T.
    (c) F.
    (d) F.
    (e) T.
    The prodromal symptoms are those symptoms which may
    have preceded the onset of psychosis by weeks or months.
    They include loss of interest in work, social activities,
    personal appearance and hygiene, together with generalized
    anxiety and mild degrees of depression and preoccupation.

37. (a) F.
    (b) F.
    (c) T. It can occur with migraine or epilepsy
    (d) F.
    (e) T.
    Autoscopy is an experience where one's own body image is
    perceived as being projected in external visual space. It is
    also known as the 'doppelgänger phenomenon'.

38. (a) F. When evoked potentials are recorded only one stimulus in one sensory modality is presented repeatedly.
    (b) T.
    (c) F. Early potentials are those that are recorded 50–80 ms post stimulus. P300 is a late positive potential that occurs 300 ms post stimulus.
    (d) F. Although a reduced amplitude of P300 has been found in some studies.
    (e) T. Early potentials on the other hand reflect activity in the primary sensory afferent pathways.

39. (a) T.
    (b) T.
    (c) T.
    (d) F.
    (e) T. Bowlby considered this to be a source of persistent anxiety.

40. (a) T.
    (b) T.
    (c) T.
    (d) T.
    (e) F.

41. (a) F. Reuptake into the presynaptic nerve terminal is a major mechanism for the active termination of neurotransmitter effects.
    (b) T.
    (c) T. They play a role, with reduced expression of messenger RNA for some receptors, following chronic treatment with agonists.
    (d) F.
    (e) T. This is manifested as a reduction in agonist response. Several processes underlie receptor adaptation.

42. (a) F.
    (b) T.
    (c) F.
    (d) F. Functional analysis is a detailed examination of the precise circumstances surrounding problem behaviour but this does not include a psychotic perceptual experience like a hallucination.
    (e) T. This includes a list of the possible reinforcers that maintain the behaviour.

43. (a) T.
    (b) T.
    (c) T.
    (d) T.
    (e) F.
    If, after a routine examination of the cognitive state, the presence of an organic cerebral disorder is suspected, an extended evaluation is necessary.

44. (a) T.
    (b) F.
    (c) F.
    (d) F.
    (e) T.
    In circumstantiality, thinking is slowed down by trivial details but it is goal directed, whereas in tangentiality thinking the goal is never reached as thinking goes off into another direction.

45. (a) T.
    (b) F. The opening of the Na^+ channels leads to an inward flow of the ions leading to depolarization.
    (c) F. The action potential lasts from 0.1 to 0.2 ms.
    (d) T.
    (e) F. Hyperpolarization is the result of inward flow of Cl^+ ions and an outward flow of K^+ ions.

46. (a) F. Pressure of speech refers to the amount of speech produced, whereas in flight of ideas the train of thoughts changes from one subject to another.
    (b) T.
    (c) F. Dysphoria is an unpleasant mood, while anhedonia means an inability to enjoy.
    (d) T. 'Made' action is a specific example of a delusion of control.
    (e) F. The terms perseveration and confabulation have been explained elsewhere in the book.

47. (a) F.
    (b) F. It was described by D. W. Winnicott.
    (c) T.
    (d) F.
    (e) T.
    Transitional objects form an important aspect of object relations theory, which deals with the involvement of the ego with reality. Transitional objects help the child to gradually move towards the acceptance of objective reality.

48. (a) F.
    (b) F.
    (c) F.
    (d) F.
    (e) F.
    Reversible inhibitors of MAO A (RIMA) do not have the 'cheese reaction' described for the older generation of monoamine oxidase inhibitors and do not have the same restrictions, although it is still prudent not to indulge excessively in tyramine-containing products.

49. (a) T. Learning that occurs by observing others is called observational learning and is a very important form of learning in infancy and childhood.
    (b) T. Modelling uses the principle of observational learning therapeutically and is an effective treatment for phobias wherein a fearless approach to a phobic situation is useful in motivating the patient to attempt to confront their phobias.
    (c) T.
    (d) F. Respondent learning is the same as classical conditioning.
    (e) T.

50. (a) T.
    (b) F.
    (c) T.
    (d) F.
    (e) T.
    Second messengers mediate an intracellular biological response following action on the cell by an extracellular first messenger.

GUIDELINES FOR THE CLINICAL EXAMINATION

The examination

The clinical examination is considered by the Royal College of Psychiatrists of the UK to be of special importance in the MRCPsych Part I examination. The candidate must obtain a pass mark in this examination in order to obtain an overall success in the whole examination, regardless of achievement in the MCQ paper. The candidate is allowed to interview the patient for 50 minutes; this is followed by a further 10 minutes to recollect thoughts and prepare for the interview with the examiners.

The clinical examination tests the basic skills of clinical assessment, which consists of psychiatric history, mental state examination, interviewing skills, role of aetiological factors, relevance of physical and psychological investigations and physical examination. It does *not* include management and prognosis of the case.

Psychiatric history

- Patient's age, sex, marital status, area of residence.
- Presenting complaints.
- Family history.
- Personal history
- Premorbid/previous personality.
- Previous medical history.
- Previous psychiatric history.
- Social history (including composition of household).
- History of presenting complaints.
- Present functioning: sleep, appetite, weight, daily routines.

The order of eliciting and/or presenting the psychiatric history may be varied. Cross references are important. The candidates are not expected to show evidence of detailed theoretical knowledge such as disease incidence in relatives, detailed biochemical theories of disease, theories of psychological development etc.

Mental state examination

– General appearance and behaviour.
– Talk: amount, flow and form.
– Thought content.
– Mood.
– Abnormal beliefs, delusions.
– Disorders of perception.
– Obsessional and compulsive phenomena.
– Cognitive function.
– Judgement.
– General knowledge.
– Insight: attitudes to illness and its treatment.

Candidates are expected to be aware of the definitions in both descriptive and dynamic psychopathology. They should show their knowledge of variations in the manifestation of psychiatric symptoms.

Interview with the examiners

Examiners work in pairs and do not require written material of the clinical examination. The interview with the examiners will occupy about 30 minutes which is divided into three parts of 10 minutes each. However, the examiners will use their discretion in deciding how much of this allotted time should be devoted to each part of the examination. This may depend on the features of the patient, and on the candidates. The following rough guide should be borne in mind:

10 minutes   The candidate to give an outline of the psychiatric history, to describe the mental state, and to give some comments on his/her interview with the patient.

10 minutes   The candidate to interview the patient in the presence of the examiners. The candidate will normally be asked to elicit certain aspects of the history or mental state.

10 minutes   Assessment of candidate's interpretation of the information obtained, and regard to any further investigations that might be useful in the given patient.

The assessment of the candidate's performance in the clinical examination is based on the following:

1. The factual information, i.e. psychiatric history elicited.

2. The mental state examination.

3. Observation of the candidate by the examiners – this includes what questions the candidate asks; how they are asked; the manifest quality of the therapeutic relationship and rapport with the patient; whether the candidate is tactful, considerate, sensitive, empathic, self-controlled, self-aware, objective, self-confident and safe. It also includes whether the candidate listens appropriately, allows the patient to talk, and is able to exercise sensitive control over the interview.

4. The candidate's appraisal of the diagnosis, differential diagnosis, aetiology, physical aspects of the case, further information required and patient's insight into his or her illness.

5. Style of presentation and delivery of the information.

PRACTICAL TIPS

Preparation for the examination

1. The examination is concerned with measuring your competency to assess patients with or without supervision.
2. There is no substitute for good clinical work and repeated practise with senior colleagues.
3. Ideally, the preparation should start from the beginning of the training.
4. Be aware of common and uncommon diagnostic categories, their most important features, differential diagnosis and treatment aspects.
5. Practise on patients suffering from diseases in major diagnostic categories.
6. Develop a list of stock questions on major diagnostic categories.
7. Establish good understanding of ICD10, DSMIIIR and DSMIV.
8. Be aware of recent college reports, college statements, government papers and important articles in leading psychiatric and medical journals.
9. A thorough history taking and mental state examination will ensure that you do not miss the relevant issues in the case.
10. Making a correct diagnosis will not necessarily ensure that you pass the examination, but a critical appraisal of the patient's clinical problems is very important.
11. Practise will probably allow you to anticipate relevant questions in the examination.

Taking the clinical examination

1. Ask the patient by what name (ie surname or first name) you should address him or her.

2. Explain the purpose of the patient's involvement in the examination.

3. Introduce the patient to the examiners. Arrange chairs in a position which allows you good eye contact with the patient. At the end of the interview (in the presence of the examiners), see the patient off and thank him or her for co-operating.

4. During the 50-minute interview with the patient, start with open-ended and less demanding questions and work your way up. If you notice that the patient is getting irritable, impatient or annoyed, change the questions or take a break from your enquiry.

5. Pay due attention to the physical examination. It is no good saying that you did not have time to perform it. Be prepared to explain what you would be looking for in the patient, eg pulse, blood pressure, optic fundi, extra-pyramidal signs, thyroid gland, focal neurological signs, etc.

6. The examiners will remind you about the format of the examination. They may use various ways to ask you about the patient, eg
   'Tell us about your patient'
   'Present your case'
   'Give us the assessment of your patient'
   'Give us a brief summary of your patient'.

7. Try to present your assessment from your memory rather than with constant reference to your handwritten notes.

8. Try to be confident and 'lucid.

9. Make use of relevant evidence from the literature to support your arguments.

10. The examiners will ask to explore or elicit a few relevant features of the patient's mental state, or the clinical history; eg obsessional features, mood, psychotic symptoms, thought content, insight, cognitive functions, premorbid personality, a typical drinking day, a typical anorexic/bulimic day, suicidal risk. etc. Occasionally you may be asked to perform a brief neurological examination.

11. Write down the questions to be asked of the patient if you can't remember, as your anxiety level is likely to be high. If you do not understand any of the questions, ask the examiners to clarify them.

    The examiners are looking for therapeutic rapport, sensitivity and empathy, and will pose a selection of questions during the interview with the patient in their presence.

12. If you cannot reach a diagnosis, be prepared to discuss the case in terms of differential diagnosis in order of priority.

13. Try not to shoot yourself in the foot. Looking too anxious and nervous may result in an unwarranted disadvantage.

FURTHER READING

Psychopathology

1. Beck, A. T. (1987) Cognitive models of depression. *Journal of Cognitive Psychotherapy*, 1:5–37.
2. Beck, A. T. and Emery, G. (1985) *Anxiety Disorders and Phobias: a Cognitive Perspective*, New York: Basic Books.
3. Brown, D. and Peddar, J. (1979) *An Introduction to Psychotherapy. An Outline of Psychodynamic Principles and Practice*, London: Tavistock Publications.
4. Gabbard, G. O. (1990) *Psychodynamic Psychiatry in Clinical Practice*, Washington, DC: American Psychiatric Press.
5. Hamilton, M. (1981) *Fish's Clinical Psychopathology. Signs and Symptoms in Psychiatry*, Bristol: John Wright and Sons.
6. Holmes, J. (ed.) (1991) *Textbook of Psychotherapy in Psychiatric Practice*, Edinburgh: Churchill Livingstone.
7. Maxwell H. (ed.) (1991) *An Outline of Psychotherapy for Trainee Psychiatrists, Medical Students and Practitioners*, 2nd edn, London and New Jersey: Whurr Publishers.
8. Murdoch, D. and Barker, P. (1991) *Basic Behaviour Therapy*, Oxford: Blackwell Scientific Publications.
9. Perris, C., Blackburn, I. M. and Perris, H. (eds) (1988) *Cognitive Psychotherapy: Theory and Practice*, Heidelberg: Springer-Verlag.
10. Rycroft, C. (1972) *A Critical Dictionary of Psychoanalysis*, Harmondsworth: Penguin.
11. Scott, J. Williams, J. M. G. and Beck, A. T. (eds) (1992) *Cognitive Therapy in Clinical Practice*, London and New York: Routledge.
12. Sims, A. (1995) *Symptoms in the Mind. An Introduction to Descriptive Psychopathology*, 2nd edn, London: Baillière Tindall.
13. Snaith, P. C. (1991) *Clinical Neurosis*, Oxford: Oxford University Press.

Classification of psychiatric disorders

1. American Psychiatric Association (1987) *Diagnostic and Statistical Manual of Mental Disorders*, 3rd edn, revised, Washington DC: American Psychiatric Association.
2. American Psychiatric Association (1994) *Diagnostic and Statistical Manual of Mental Disorders*, 4th edn, Washington DC: American Psychiatric Association.
3. Foulds, G. A. (1976) *The Hierarchical Nature of Personal Illness*, London: Academic Press.
4. Spitzer, R. L., Endicott, J. and Robins, E. (1978) Research diagnostic criteria: Rationale and reliability. *Archives of General Psychiatry*, **35**: 773–782.
5. World Health Organization (1992) *ICD-10: The ICD-10 Classification of Mental and Behavioural Disorders*, Geneva: World Health Organization.

Methods of clinical assessment

(History-taking, mental state examination, process of diagnosis, aetiological factors of psychiatric disorders)
1. Gelder, M., Gath, D. and Mayou, R. (1993) *Oxford Textbook of Psychiatry*, Oxford: Oxford Medical Publications, Oxford University Press.
2. Kendell, R. E. and Zealley, A. M. (eds) (1993) *Companion to Psychiatric Studies*, 5th edn, Edinburgh: Churchill Livingstone.
3. Leff, J. P. and Isaacs, A. D. (1990) *Psychiatric Examination in Clinical Practice*, London: Blackwell Scientific Publications.
4. Paykel, E. (ed.) (1992) *Handbook of Affective Disorders*, Edinburgh: Churchill Livingstone.
5. Shea, S. C. (1988) *Psychiatric Interviewing. The Art of Understanding*, Philadelphia: W. B. Saunders Company, Harcourt Brace Jovanovich.

Basic clinical psychopharmacology

1. King, D. (1993) *Seminars in Psychopharmacology*, College Seminar Series, Gaskell: Royal College of Psychiatrists.
2. Silverstone, T. and Turner, P. (1991) *Drug Treatment in Psychiatry*, London and New York: Routledge.

Neurosciences and neurological examination

1. Lishman, W. A. (1987) *Organic Psychiatry*, 2nd edn, London: Blackwell Scientific Publications.
2. Morgan, G. and Butler, S. (eds) (1993) *Seminars in Basic Neurosciences*, College Seminar Series, Gaskell: Royal College of Psychiatrists.
3. Puri, B. K. and Tyrer, P. J. (1992) *Sciences Basic to Psychiatry*, Edinburgh: Churchill Livingstone.

INDEX